Praise for *Tai Chi Concepts and Experin*

"With a lifetime of commitment to deep study and practice, diligent teaching, and the promotion of the martial arts, Robert Chuckrow, Ph.D., sets an example of how to grow your personal practice through contributing to the greater martial arts community. Now, through this book, he has demonstrated a determination and commitment to understanding the depth of martial arts practice."

> — Grandmaster Sam F.S. Chin, Founder of Zhong Xin Dao, Gatekeeper of I Liq Chuan, Author of *I Liq Chuan—Martial Art of Awareness, I Liq Chuan System Guide* and nearly 30 DVDs, Honorary Professor Emeritus.

"It's my great pleasure to recommend this latest book on Tai Chi by my friend and Tai Chi classmate, Dr. Chuckrow, a Tai Chi devotee who never stops studying and learning. As a Western scientist, he delves deeply into the esoteric jargon, principles, and teachings of Tai Chi and reinterprets them for Westerners."

> — Lawrence Galante, Ph.D., author of *Tai Chi: the Supreme Ultimate, Energy Healing*; Director of The Center for Holistic Arts, NYC; Professor at State University of New York.

"Author Robert Chuckrow offers his enlightening wisdom and educated perspective on the paradoxes of Tai Chi in his latest work. Through [his] brilliant research, Chuckrow resolves so many nagging questions that all beginners have and offers many new tools for instructors to share this venerated art. It's a must-read work for Tai Chi practitioners of every level, not to be missed."

> — Gene Ching, 32nd generation disciple of the Shaolin Temple, author of *Shaolin Trips*, publisher of *Kung Fu Magazine*, former publisher of *Kung Fu Tai Chi*, weapons expert for El Rey Network's original TV show, *Man at Arms: Art of War*.

"Robert Chuckrow is a teacher and scientist who comprehends and synthesizes what he learns and then shares it for the benefit of others. He couples his knowledge of physics with his Tai-Chi skills, and the result enables the reader to understand this art more clearly than they could from studying translations of ancient cryptic Chinese sayings.

"People learn Tai Chi for different reasons—some for health, some for self-defense, and others for philosophical or spiritual reasons. And some do Tai Chi for years without understanding much of what they do, which will still make them healthier and more sensitive to the world around them. But they will miss the wondrous benefits that a deeper study will offer. This book will take you further along this path."

— Ken Van Sickle, Professor Emeritus at NYU, Tai Chi master in the lineage of Cheng Man-ch'ing, third-dan black belt in karate under Peter Urban, author of *Ken Van Sickle Photography*.

"Robert Chuckrow's new book offers tremendous insights into the physical, spiritual, and healing aspects of Tai Chi. His discussion of natural movement and expansive strength is enlightening and well-referenced. Dr. Chuckrow encourages readers to perform the experiments he sets forth in order to experience for themselves the sensations and therapeutic benefits of expansive strength. He promotes critical thinking, reviews historical perspectives, and clarifies classical teachings. This book will enhance the practice of any student of this ancient and powerful art."

— Dr. Catherine Kurosu, MD, L.Ac. Co-author of the *True Wellness* book series.

"I was immediately impressed with Robert Chuckrow's approach to the soft-style arts. In the beginning of the book, Dr. Chuckrow's discussion of expansive strength versus contractive strength was immediately useful to me in my daily practice. Every chapter that followed presented new insights and ideas that I had not considered before, as well as exercises and experiments that helped me experience them directly."

— Master Joe Varady, M.Ed., Rokudan, author of *The Art and Science of Staff Fighting* and *The Art and Science of Stick Fighting*.

"With chapters on expansive strength, swimming on land, rooting and redirecting, natural movement, relaxation and timing, plus many more, this book is a guide to learning, practicing and better understanding Tai Chi. Dr. Chuckrow, an experienced Tai Chi practitioner and teacher, writes with the same attention to detail as when he teaches physics. In this book, he turns difficult, archaic Chinese sayings into clear and easy-to-understand English by using simple and practical exercises to get his meaning across."

— Mario Napoli, Tai Chi practitioner since 1988, black belt in karate and judo, All-China National Push-Hands Champion in Chen Village competition, 1988.

"As a physicist, Chuckrow offers the unique perspective of a scientific analysis of the practice of Tai Chi. As a student of Cheng Man-ching, his years of explorations and discoveries have yielded deep insights into this extraordinary art."

— Barry Strugatz, filmmaker, director of the
documentary *The Professor: Tai Chi's Journey West*.

"This book is an excellent interpretation of Tai Chi Classics, which has been written through the centuries by the highest-level Tai Chi masters. Dr. Chuckrow has put forth these ideas and concepts in simple, easy-to-understand English. He explains these concepts using modern scientific principles of physics and the mechanics of human movement. He gives many examples and experiments to help students understand the principles of Tai Chi in a new light. This book is a must-read for all serious students of Tai Chi."

— Leonard Antonucci, taekwondo fifth-degree black
belt, professor of health sciences, Long Island
University, NY (retired).

"Reading Professor Chuckrow's book proves that efficient movement is efficient movement, no matter if it's done in Tai Chi or Kodokan Judo. One comment that Professor Chuckrow made was '. . . wasteful movement is unnatural.' This, in a nutshell, also describes what we do in judo. Another nugget of practical wisdom is, ...moving efficiently, using the smallest possible movements, provides an advantage.' One would think that this came out of a judo book—again, proving that efficient movement is efficient movement, no matter the context."

— Steve Scott, author of *The Judo Advantage*, *The Juji
Gatame Encyclopedia*, *The Sambo Encyclopedia*, and
other books.

"This book has reignited my passion to further explore the art [of Tai Chi]."

— Peter Doherty, Master Trainer of Corrective
Exercise, twenty-eight years studying martial arts,
black belt in Karate.

"Brilliant! A high-level teacher of both Tai Chi Chuan and physics takes us along on his own fifty-year exploration into the very heart of China's most respected 'internal martial art,' challenging us each step of the way to deepen our own understanding of this marvelous practice. [This] is a book that every Tai Chi practitioner—and beyond that, every martial artist—should read, cogitate upon, and keep for life-long reference."

— Myles Angus MacVane, Tai Chi Chuan expert.

"The mysteries of the Chinese martial art Tai Chi are illuminated with the help of science in this primer.

"Chuckrow—the author of *Tai Chi Dynamics* (2008), a physicist, and a Tai Chi instructor— addresses the seemingly contradictory teachings of the masters of this martial art, like the admonition to use "no strength" in practicing it, and interprets them in light of Western physics and biology. His main idea is the concept of "expansive strength," a kind of "hydraulic pressure" in which "bodily tissues can actively expand under the action of bioelectrical stimulation." Expansive strength, he contends, is better than ordinary strength through muscle contractions because it doesn't create metabolic waste products or telegraph one's intentions to attackers. He goes on to apply more physics—explained in plain English, with the math tucked away in the appendix—to Tai Chi problems, like the niceties of maintaining one's balance in a pushing match. ("If an opponent A exerts a force F on me, according to Newton's third law, I automatically exert the same force F on A in the opposite direction....In order to remain in balance, A must arrange things so that the total frictional force of the floor on his feet exerts a force that is opposite to the force I am exerting on him.") Much of the intricate book explores Tai Chi's preoccupation with an exhaustive, even eye-glazing analysis of rudimentary bodily acts, such as taking a step—"As the knee k starts to arc forward, the lower leg lags behind, swinging backward relative to the upper leg; (b) the knee stops, and the lower leg swings forward past (c) to (d); (d) the lower leg has freely swung forward into a position with the heel just touching the ground"—or sitting down. ("True Tai-Chi practitioners lower themselves slowly and first contact the chair without any commitment. Then, they mindfully transfer weight until it is safe to commit it fully.") Physiologists may scratch their heads at Chuckrow's notion of expansive strength, but otherwise his explications of the fundamental laws of natural motion, complete with diagrams, are written in reasonably clear, if involved, prose. Tai chi students will gain from the author a deep theoretical grounding in the discipline's basic approach to movement along with a wealth of useful exercises to help them practice it.

"This informative introduction to Tai Chi combines extensive discussions of principles with hands-on techniques."

— KIRKUS Reviews

Tai Chi Concepts and Experiments

Tai Chi Concepts and Experiments

Hidden Strength, Natural Movement, and Timing

Robert Chuckrow, Ph.D.

YMAA Publication Center
Wolfeboro, NH USA

YMAA Publication Center, Inc.
PO Box 480
Wolfeboro, NH 03894
800 669-8892 • www.ymaa.com • info@ymaa.com
ISBN: 9781594397417 (print) • ISBN: 9781594397424 (ebook)
This book set in Adobe Garamond and Frutiger

20200401

Publisher's Cataloging in Publication

Names: Chuckrow, Robert, author, illustrator.

Title: Tai chi concepts and experiments : hidden strength, natural movement, and timing / Robert Chuckrow ; illustrated by the author.

Description: Wolfeboro, NH USA : YMAA Publication Center, [2021] | Includes bibliographical references and index.

Identifiers: ISBN: 9781594397417 | 9781594397424 (ebook) | LCCN: 2021930021

Subjects: LCSH: Tai chi--Physiological aspects. | Physiology, Experimental. | Stretching exercises. | Muscle strength. | Movement, Psychology of. | Motor ability--Physiological aspects. | Reaction time. | Qi (Chinese philosophy) | Spirituality. | Mind and body. | BISAC: HEALTH & FITNESS / Exercise / Stretching. | HEALTH & FITNESS / Tai Chi. | BODY, MIND & SPIRIT / Healing / Energy (Qigong, Reiki, Polarity) | SCIENCE / Life Sciences / Human Anatomy & Physiology. | SPORTS & RECREATION / Martial Arts / General. | SPORTS & RECREATION / Health & Safety.

Classification: LCC: GV504 .C58 2021 | DDC: 613.7/148--dc23

Printed in Canada.

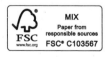

Dedication

To Elaine Summers and Sam Chin Fan-siong, from whom
I received an understanding of expansive strength.

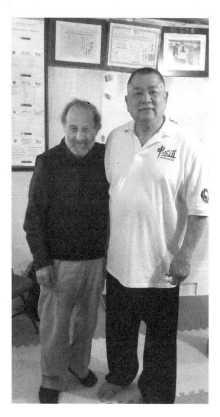

The author (left) and Sam Chin Fan-siong (right).
(Photo by Kenneth Van Sickle)

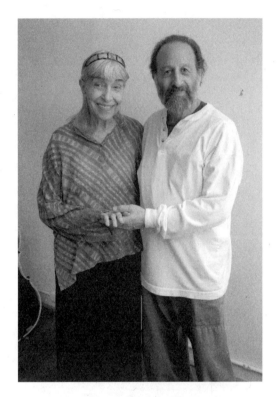

Elaine Summers and the author in 2007.
(Photo by Kenneth Van Sickle)

CONTENTS

AUTHOR'S NOTE

Wherever elementary physics is employed in treating certain material, an intuitive explanation of that material is also provided for readers unfamiliar with physics. Throughout, I have striven to minimize repetition of material covered in my other books and, when possible, to use entirely new material or a new way of presenting it. In some cases, however, I have revisited prior material with a new perspective.

Every effort has been made to be accurate and helpful. I have experienced *for myself* the truth of what I have written here. However, there may be typographical errors or mistakes in content, or some of the content may not be applicable to everyone. It is my wish that the reader exercise skepticism and caution in applying the information and ideas herein. The purpose of any controversial parts of this book is to stimulate the reader's thinking rather than to serve as an ultimate source of information.

The book is sold with the understanding that neither the author nor publisher is engaged in rendering medical or other advice. If medical advice or other expert assistance is required, the services of a competent health-care professional should be sought. Therefore, neither the author nor publisher shall be held liable or responsible for any harm to anyone from the direct or indirect application of the knowledge or ideas expressed herein.

The pinyin transliteration of Chinese words is used throughout this work, but names of people have been retained in Wade-Giles. For consistency, the Wade-Giles transliterations that occur in older quoted material have been changed to pinyin.

In Wade-Giles, the letter(s) immediately before the apostrophe are not voiced, and the absence of an apostrophe signifies that those letters are voiced. For example, the letter *T* in *T'ai* is pronounced as the *t* in *tar* (*t* not voiced), and the *T* in *Tao* is pronounced as the *d* in *doubt* (*t* is voiced). Similarly, the *ch* in *Chi* is pronounced as the *jee* in *jeep* (*ch* voiced), and the *ch* in *ch'i* is pronounced as the *ch* in *cheap* (not voiced).

Asian words are italicized except for names of people and familiar arts (e.g., Cheng Man-ch'ing and Taijiquan).

The following table lists some correspondences between the two forms of transliteration:[1]

Wade-Giles	Pinyin
T'ai-Chi Ch'uan	Taijiquan
ch'i	*qi*
Ch'i Kung	Qigong
p'eng	*peng*
k'ua	*kua*
p'i p'a	*pipa*

---

1. For a more-complete list of pinyin/Wade-Giles conversions, see http://library.ust.hk/guides/opac/conversion-tables.html.

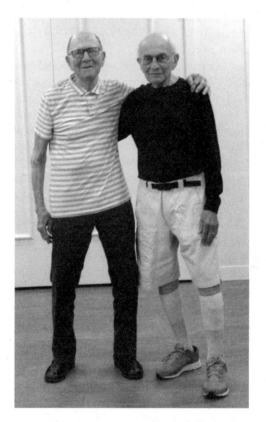

Two of the author's Taiji students (William Rakower, left, and Myron Gordon, right). Both were ninety-nine years of age when the photo was taken. Both have since reached one hundred.

INTRODUCTION

Why I Wrote This Book

Over the half-century that I have studied Taiji, I have found that explanations of certain essential elements of the art are either insufficiently clear or absent. Two such elements are (1) the cultivation of expansive strength, which does not originate from nerve impulses producing contraction of muscle fibers but from a different action, and (2) the optimal timing of movement from the legs, to the hips, and out to the arms. I am concerned that these two essential elements will be forever lost to the majority of Taiji practitioners, especially those of the Yang style.

The writings of the highest-level masters over centuries are contained in the Taiji Classics. These writings emphasize the importance of releasing ordinary strength until it is at a minimum but also emphasize cultivating a kind of strength described as "iron wrapped in cotton." On the one hand, the body must be so free of tension that the slightest touch will set the body into motion. On the other hand, the whole body must be able to manifest substantial strength in all directions—even while doing the Taiji form. These two ideas seem contradictory.

Over the decades, I have come to understand that there is no contradiction and that there are two different kinds of strength, contractive and expansive. It now makes perfect sense that relinquishing contractive strength is essential to achieving expansive strength. That idea is confirmed by what I have observed in my teachers and what is expressed in the Taiji Classics.

A main goal in writing this book is to resolve the seeming strength/no-strength contradiction and enable the reader to achieve expansive strength. Another goal is to clarify the optimal timing of the turning of the trunk of the body relative to that of the arms to maximize the transfer of movement from the feet, to the body, to the arms, and to provide ways of recognizing and then achieving this timing.

Whereas some of my analysis involves the application of basic physics, the reader need not know any physics to gain the desired understanding—the final conclusions are simply and clearly stated, intuitive examples are given, and various experiments are provided for the reader to try. Readers who are interested in the rigorous physics derivations will find them in the appendices.

Contents Overview

The first chapter addresses the concept of relaxation. The next two chapters explore the idea of expansive strength. Experiments that the reader can apply for experiencing such strength are provided, and physiological arguments are advanced. We then show the advantages of expansive strength, its healing aspects and protocols, and how it enters into the Taiji movements.

Two other chapters cover balance and rooting. Several chapters address and clarify how to achieve the most relaxed and natural timing of movement regardless of speed. A chapter is provided on clarifying Cheng Man-ch'ing's treatise on the physics of Taiji. Other chapters will address self-cultivation and maximizing progress in studying Taiji.

Who Should Read This Book

Teachers and advanced practitioners of Taiji will find that this book contains clear explanations and perspectives of essential elements infrequently—if ever—available. Exposure to ideas that might conflict with or are absent from their Taiji or other training will provide much food for thought and accelerate their progress.

Practitioners with some experience should find that the ideas presented herein will enhance their understanding.

Finally, beginners will struggle to understand some of the ideas presented, but for many the exposure should pay off in the future.

Chapter 1
"Relax"

Cheng Man-ch'ing

I started my study of Taiji in 1970 with Professor Cheng Man-ch'ing (1902–1975) at the T'ai-Chi Ch'uan Association at 211 Canal Street, New York City. I was then thirty-three years of age and am now eighty-four.

At that time, I had almost no idea what Taiji was. All I knew was that I was very high-strung and uncoordinated, and after my initial skepticism, Taiji appeared to be a solution to these issues.

Professor Cheng spoke and understood only Mandarin, of which I knew not even one word. So everything I asked him was translated into Mandarin, and then Professor Cheng's answers in Mandarin were translated back into English. Professor Cheng also communicated silently, using various gestures.

One of the first things I was repeatedly told in class was to relax. In fact, "relax" was the reply to most questions my classmates and I asked.

As I learned to relax, I saw how doing so helped everything I did. I started to recognize all of the unnecessary tension I was applying to using a table saw, practicing the harpsichord, washing dishes, driving my car, and even getting out of bed in the morning.

Yang Cheng-fu

Cheng Man-ch'ing was an inner student of Yang Cheng-fu (1883–1936), who was considered to be one of the top-ten Chinese martial artists of the 20th century—quite an accomplishment considering the millions of high-level martial artists in China during that century.

In class, Professor Cheng said that *relax* (*song*) was the main word used by Yang. Here are Professor Cheng's words to that effect:

Relax (*song*). My teacher must have repeated these words many times each day. "Relax! Relax! Relax completely! The whole body should completely relax!" Otherwise he said, "Not relaxed. Not relaxed. If you are not relaxed, then you are like a punching bag."[1]

"If you are not relaxed, then you are like a punching bag" can perhaps be interpreted as follows: as soon as you stiffen when embroiled in a real fight with a high-level Taijiquan practitioner who is adept at using softness, that is when you will get hit.

The Meaning of *Relax*

It took time for me to learn that *relax* is routinely used as an English translation for the Chinese word *song*. The character for *song* (see Fig. 1-1) includes a pine tree (lower part) and hair (upper part). The drooping branches and hair suggest letting the musculature relax to the point of having the nonexistent strength of hair. *Relax*, however, implies letting go totally, which is one aspect of *song*. But *song* also has a supportive aspect (suggested by the trunk of the tree). The idea is that when in a state of *song*, your skeleton supplies an upward support to the body even though the musculature is drooping. So when the word *relax* is used in Taiji, it is understood that the muscles are releasing, but the integrity and optimal alignment of the skeleton is maintained.

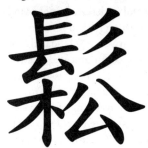

Fig. 1-1. The character for *song*, which is often translated into English as *relax*. The character includes a pine tree (lower part) and hair (upper part).

---

1. Cheng Man-ch'ing, *Cheng Tzu's Thirteen Treatises on T'ai Chi Ch'uan*, tr. Benjamin Pang Jen Lo and Martin Inn (Berkeley, CA: North Atlantic Books, 1981), 88.

Attaining *Song*

> **Experiment 1-1.** Stand with your feet parallel, a comfortable distance apart. Release all tension in your body. Recreate the heavy feeling you get after a hot bath—especially when you let the water drain out while you recline in the tub. Release your eyes (liquefy your eyeballs and feel them pooling in their sockets). Release your temples, nasal passages, jaw, tongue, throat, shoulders, back, arms, chest, abdomen, lower abdomen, and even your legs. Feel the heaviness of everything hanging from and supported by your skeleton. Do not let your head droop but extend its top upward without contracting your neck muscles.

The Importance of Releasing Tension in Doing Taiji Movement Stability (Root)

Another aspect of *song* is "root." That is, by attaining a state of *song*, your center of gravity is low, and you are "rooted" to the ground similarly to a tree.

> **Experiment 1-2.** Stand with your feet parallel, a comfortable distance apart. Release all tension in your body. Recreate the heavy feeling you get after a hot bath. Release everything mentioned in Experiment 1-1. Feel how stable you are. Then tense your chest. Feel your center of mass rise and your stability decrease.

> **Experiment 1-3.** Stand in a 70-30 stance (see Fig. 1-2). Have a partner push you backward. Then tense your upper body and notice how much easier it is for your partner to move you. Then release everything downward; have your partner push you again with the same strength as before and observe any increase in stability.

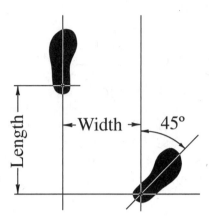

Fig. 1-2. The positioning of the feet in a 70-30 stance. The rear foot is at 45° to the direction of the stance and bears 30 percent of the weight of the body. The feet are a shoulder width apart. To test this width, rotate your rear foot inward on its heel until its centerline is parallel to that of your forward foot. The separation of these two centerlines should be equal to the distance between your shoulder joints. To test the length, shift your weight 100 percent onto your rear leg, letting your forward leg slide backward until it stops. Any backward movement means that when you originally stepped into that stance, you overreached that foot and prematurely committed your weight.

Health

Professor Cheng reminded us that our distant ancestors walked on all fours, with their midsections hanging from their spines. Every step provided healthful movement of organs, glands, and other bodily tissues. The movement also promoted free flow of blood, with its transport of oxygen and nutrients into cells and waste products out. Becoming upright provided enormous developmental value. But we paid a health price by having our organs stacked one upon the other, with little freedom to move or receive nutritive and cleansing effects. Of course, there is no turning back, but by relaxing and doing healthful movement, we can mitigate some of the harmful effects.

Spirituality

Song also has a spiritual aspect. By learning to release unneeded physical tension, we are paving the way for also releasing wrong thinking and the frequent overstepping of bounds of our emotional systems. However, walking that path requires sustained vigilance, critical but objective self-observation, and consistent work. Success is definitely not automatic.

Push-Hands

After a year of learning Professor Cheng's Taiji form, I was allowed to start learning push-hands, a two-person exercise wherein each participant tries to uproot the other by using the Taiji principles. Here too, we were told not to use any strength and relax completely. The question was how it could be possible to push someone without using strength. When Professor Cheng would push a student, he always did so by first touching him or her. Whenever he pushed me, I was amazed by his wonderful precision and how little force it took for him to send me flying, but still, some strength was needed.

A Seeming Contradiction

Because I saw how much value Taiji study and practice provided, I overlooked the glaring impossibility of doing the movements by using zero strength and simply devoted myself to moving in the most relaxed manner possible.

There was, however, one unanswered question: How could I lift an arm or even move a finger without using any strength? Of course, I knew that these actions could be done more efficiently by letting go of all *unnecessary* strength. Yet my classmates and I were repeatedly told to do the Taiji movements without using *any* strength. Using no strength was an obvious impossibility, but the senior students insisted that it was possible.

I could understand the possibility that what was really meant was to reduce the amount of strength used to a bare minimum and that I should not take "use no strength" literally. But Taijiquan originated in China as a martial art hundreds of years ago and was the top martial art for a long time. The idea that Taiji training involves learning to use minimal strength seems antithetical to its martial aspect. In the words of Stanley Israel (1942–1999), an accomplished martial artist and a senior student at Professor Cheng's school, "It is impossible for there to be a martial art that does not use some sort of strength."

As mentioned earlier, the character for *song* involves a pine tree, with its strong central trunk and downward-hanging branches (Fig. 1-1). The trunk can be thought of as *yang* (reaching upward) and the hanging branches as *yin*. In the context of Taiji movement, however, the trunk can also be thought of as *yin*—it is supportive and rooted in the earth, with no power for producing expansive movement. Such movement was exhibited and emphasized by my later teachers, Harvey Sober and Sam Chin, and required by a martial art. So a *yang* counterpart to *song* is required in order to balance *yin* and *yang*.

Shedding Some Light on the No-Strength Paradox

Yang Cheng-fu, whose main admonition was to relax, also said:

> Taiji is the art of concealing hardness within softness.[2]

Additionally, Yang said:

> The Taiji Classics say, "When you are extremely soft, then you become extremely hard and strong." Someone who has extremely good Taijiquan *gongfu* has arms like iron wrapped in cotton, and the weight is very heavy.[3]

In addition to advising us to relax, Professor Cheng talked about what he called "swimming on land" (discussed in Chapter 3) and advised "feeling" the air to have the resistance of water.[4,5] He also said, "As you make greater progress, the air will not only feel heavier than water, it will feel like iron."[6] This assertion suggests that practicing swimming on land can lead to the cultivation of demonstrable physical strength.

The sayings of Professor Cheng, Yang Cheng-fu and the Taiji Classics imply that there is something beyond the admonition to use no strength—that there is another kind of strength and developing that strength can only occur by first releasing habitual, conventional strength.

Dr. George K. W. Ho's article in *Tai Chi Magazine*[7] is extremely helpful in clarifying that Yang Cheng-fu used the words *song kai*. The additional word, *kai* (Fig. 1-2), involves the concept of openness, activation, and expansion—beautifully expressing the *yang* counterpart needed for balancing *song!*

2. Douglas Wile, comp. and trans., *T'ai Chi Touchstones: Yang Family Secret Transmissions* (Brooklyn, NY: Sweet Ch'i Press, 1983), 3.
3. Benjamin Pang Jeng Lo, Martin Inn, Robert Amacker, and Susan Foe, eds., *The Essence of T'ai Chi Ch'uan, The Literary Tradition* (Berkeley, CA: North Atlantic Books, 1985), 87.
4. Cheng Man-ch'ing, *Tai Chi Chuan: A Simplified Method of Calisthenics for Health and Self Defense* (Berkeley, CA: North Atlantic Books, 1985),10.
5. Cheng Man-ch'ing and Robert W. Smith, *T'ai Chi: The Supreme Ultimate" Exercise for Health, Sport, and Self Defense* (Rutland, VT: Charles E. Tuttle Co., 1967), 2.
6. Cheng Man-ch'ing, *Cheng Tzu's Thirteen Treatises on T'ai Chi Ch'uan*, trans. Benjamin Pang Jen Lo and Martin Inn (Berkeley, CA: North Atlantic Books, 1981), 39.
7. Dr. George K. W. Ho, "Going beyond the Term Relaxation," *Tai Chi Magazine* 38, no. 1 (Spring 2014): 6–9.

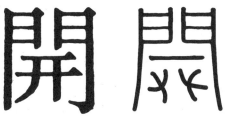

Fig. 1-3. Left, the character for *kai, to open*. The character is formed by 門, a gate and 开, a contraction of two hands and the bolt to lock the gate, shown in the old character (right), suggesting that someone is going to open the gate.[8]

Interestingly, the word *kai* can mean activate (boil water or turn on the TV) or, after a verb, indicate expansion or development (the news has spread far and wide).[9]

One of the primary objects of this book will be to show how striving to reduce the use of conventional strength can make a practitioner very strong but in a totally unconventional way. This point of view is at odds with the oft-stated idea that the strength developed is not unconventional but finely tailored conventional strength that is always kept at a minimum.

In the following pages, much will be said about *song* and how it is necessary but not sufficient for developing the kind of strength legendary in Taiji. It is important that the reader keep an open mind and not shut the door to the unconventional aspect of this art.

8. Oreste Vaccari and Enko Elsoa Vaccari, *Pictorial Chinese-Japanese Characters* (Rutland, VT: Charles E. Tuttle Co., 1950), 137.

9. Martin H. Manser, *Concise English-Chinese Chinese-English Dictionary*, 2nd ed. (Hong Kong: Oxford University Press, Hong Kong), 248–249.

Chapter 2
Expansive Strength

Is there one kind of strength that in Taiji is used in a minimal, highly trained manner? Or are there two distinctly different kinds of strength, one type being ordinary muscular contraction and the other kind not involving muscular contraction but something quite different? And if there are two kinds, are they perhaps used alternately or in unison?

We will explore the hypothesis that bodily tissues can actively expand under the action of bioelectrical stimulation. I have thought about and experimented with this hypothesis since the mid-1970s and have continued to be increasingly convinced of its truth. Until recently, the evidence was based on what I (and others) have been experiencing. Now the experiential evidence is supported by ongoing scientific research at Washington State University, led by Dr. Gerald Pollack. That research on water and its effect on cellular action identified a mechanism by which tissues can actively expand, a mechanism that corresponds closely to what I have been experiencing and describing for decades—and what others can experience if so taught.

Intention is involved in such expansion, so it might seem that electrical nerve impulses play a part. But there might also be a different, more evolutionary, and primitive biological mechanism of electrical transmission. If you watch videos of protists (single-celled, microscopic animals) moving, they devour microscopic prey, dart around as if having the intention to do so, and seem to avoid obstacles deliberately.[1] Yet they have no muscles, eyes, or known nervous systems. As we have evolved from such life forms grouping together, perhaps we retain primordial mechanisms of sensing and of changing cellular states that involve some sort of electrical transmission beyond a neurological one. Thus, the more-general term *bioelectricity* will be used hereinafter to refer

---

1. See videos of protists: https://www.youtube.com/watch?v=4aZneo5Qu4Q and https://www.youtube.com/watch?v=-8rpGbHC2Jo.

to electric potentials and currents produced by or occurring within living organisms.

First, I will explain how I was introduced to the concept of expansive strength. Next, I will provide some experiments that readers can try for exploring expansive strength. Finally, I will summarize a promising mechanism for expansive strength.

Background

I started my study of Kinetic Awareness® (KA) in 1974 under Elaine Summers (1925–2014).[2] KA is a system of natural movement and self-discovery that she originated. KA® includes the concept that muscles can actively extend. Summers called this phenomenon *extension tension*. Much of her work in analyzing bodily movement and helping injured dancers recover was based on this concept. There is great therapeutic benefit in relinquishing the contractive strength to which most of us are habituated and slowly, mindfully, and painlessly extending the tissues that are in trauma.

The reason for the therapeutic effectiveness of relaxed, mindful movement is that it promotes the flow of *qi* and blood, both of which are otherwise restricted by the contraction of muscles. Blood transports oxygen and nutrients to and waste products away from the traumatized region. Moreover, the bioelectricity resulting from such relaxed movement stimulates the absorption of beneficial substances and the release of waste products.

Decades ago, I began to realize that expansive strength was the key to what in Taiji is called *nei jin. Nei* means *internal*, and *jin* means *strength*. This realization greatly enhanced my progress in Taiji.

In 2008, I stated in *Tai Chi Dynamics* the hypothesis that muscles can actively extend.[3] I utilized that concept to explain natural and reverse breathing and also the important distinction between *nei jin* (strength arising from internal training) and *li* (untrained strength). Moreover, I applied that concept to a number of other often-elusive Taiji applications. The concept of expansive strength also served to clarify otherwise mysterious passages of the Taiji Classics. I stated then that I experienced muscular extension as hydraulic pressure wherein a change in pressure at any part of the body is transmitted to every other part of the body (bodily unification).

The Current View of Muscular Action

The following are the current views:

---

2. http://en.wikipedia.org/wiki/Elaine_Summers.

3. Robert Chuckrow, *Tai Chi Dynamics* (Wolfeboro, NH: YMAA Publication Center, 2008), 1–23.

a. Muscular action results *solely* from the contraction of muscle fibers along their length.

b. The contraction of muscle fibers is activated by neural impulses from the brain, spinal cord, or other muscles.

c. Muscles are arranged in opposing pairs.

d. The contraction of a muscle on one side causes the muscle(s) on the other side to elongate (extend).

The discussion that follows in the next section agrees with the above views except for the word *solely* in (a). Namely, we advance the hypothesis that there is an additional way in which muscles (or other tissues) elongate (or expand) other than solely by the contraction of opposing muscles. That is, we hypothesize that contraction is not the only feature of muscular action, and muscles and possibly other bodily tissues can actively produce movement through expansion.

Differences between Contractive and Expansive Strength

Expansive strength is better for sensitively doing short-range, precise excursions and for sustaining a position against an opposing force or neutralizing an incoming attack. Short-range movement is consistent with the Taiji principle that neutralizing and striking originates in the legs and "waist" and not in the arms.

> The motion should be rooted in the feet, released through the legs, controlled by the waist, and manifested through the fingers.[4]
>
> —Chang San-feng

So expansion excels for Taiji movements, which involve small excursions of all body parts in a unified manner.

> Remember, when moving, there is no place that doesn't move. When still, there is no place that isn't still.[5]
>
> —Wu Yu-hsiang (1812–1880)

The above saying can be interpreted to mean that every part of the body *actively* participates in and fully contributes to the movement of all parts. In expansive movement, the contribution of any localized part is relatively small when all parts participate in a unified manner. So the whole body can have a moderately large movement.

---

4. Benjamin Pang Jeng Lo, Martin Inn, Robert Amacker, and Susan Foe, eds., *The Essence of T'ai Chi Ch'uan, The Literary Tradition* (Berkeley, CA: North Atlantic Books, 1985), 21.

5. Lo et al., *The Essence of T'ai Chi Ch'uan*, 57.

For most tasks in daily life, contractive muscular action is appropriate. Contraction is especially good for generating large-range movement and a large amount of force for a short period of time. In Taiji movement, however, we seek to cultivate a specialized, alternative kind of relaxed, expansive strength suitable for cultivating health and, for those so inclined, for training the martial aspect of Taijiquan.

Some Experiential Evidence for Expansive Strength (Experiments You Can Do)

Trying the following experiments (some of which are described in *Tai Chi Dynamics*) should, at the very least, lead you to be skeptical of the conventional idea that expansive strength is impossible.

Note: To maximize the desired effect in each of the following explorations, it is important to:

1. Relax contractive tension of the part(s) being moved as much as possible.
2. Imagine movement while in a relaxed state without doing any actual movement, which results in neural electricity being sent from the brain and spinal cord to the part imagined.
3. Feel the state achieved in (1) and (2), and capture that feeling.
4. Only then do actual movements while recreating the feeling attained through imagination.

Experiment 2-1. Expanding Your Midsection. The ability to feel your midsection (the lower abdomen extending around to the sides, plus the back of the waist) and voluntarily expand it is important for recognizing expansion and extending it into other parts of the body. One way to recognize a modality is to refer to what you already can do, even if only involuntarily. Specifically, such expansion occurs naturally without necessarily having conscious awareness of its mechanics when you breathe. The goal is to learn to do that expansion voluntarily, independently of breathing. The following experiment involves two people, *A* and *B*.

(continued on next page)

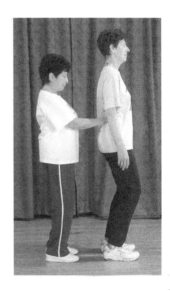

Fig. 2-1. A student testing another for expansion of the midsection.[1]

---

1. This photo was reproduced from Robert Chuckrow, *Tai Chi Dynamics*, 17.

Referring to Figure 2-1, *A* stands behind *B* and places her hands on B's waist, just below her ribs. *A* then presses inward, and B then tries to move A's hands outward by expanding her midsection to the front, sides, and rear. When *A* feels an increase in pressure on her hands, she tells *B*. Then *B* knows that she is successful and locks in the feeling so she can recreate it again. If more pressure is needed for recognition, *A* can press with the web of each hand (the part between thumb and forefinger).

Once *B* succeeds in producing a voluntary expansion of her midsection, *A* and *B* exchange roles. Afterward, participants should strive to learn to voluntarily expand all other parts of their bodies in doing Qigong and Taiji movement.

In addition to being a tool for recognizing expansion, the ability to voluntarily expand your midsection subtly—not forcibly—is essential for doing reverse breathing[6] and for unifying the entire trunk of the body.

Note: Taking a deep in-breath will automatically expand your midsection, and it is good to do that to feel what happens. But the goal here is to expand voluntarily, independently of whether you are breathing in or out.

Experiment 2-2. Opening Your Hand. Sit or stand, and relax as much as possible. Hold your arm in front of you such that your hand is relaxed and a comfortable distance from your body. Imagine that you have an expanding balloon in the palm of your hand. Remember that it is important not to do any actual movement at first. Then, very slowly open your hand a tiny amount, imagining that doing so is a result of the expanding balloon. Pay special attention to the feeling of the palm of the hand and the inside of the forearm as compared to the back of the hand and the outside of the forearm. See how open you can make your hand without losing the feeling just referred to.

Once you are familiar with the feeling of this action, now try opening your hand in the usual way by pulling it open by contracting the muscles that are connected to the back of your hand. Again, as your hand opens, pay special attention to the feeling of the palm of the hand and the inside of the forearm as compared to the back of the hand and the outside of the forearm. See how much more you can open your hand by using contraction. Pay attention to the feeling involved.

Compare the difference in feeling between the first and second ways of opening your hand, namely, expansion and contraction, respectively. Moreover, expansion results only in opening the hand somewhat but not in straightening your fingers, whereas contraction can cause your fingers to

---

6. Chuckrow, *Tai Chi Dynamics*, Ch. 2.

actually hyperextend (bend backwards). Last, compare the feeling of *qi* in the two hands for both ways. I think that you will find that expansion provides much more *qi*. Chapter 3, "Swimming on Land," has experiments for experiencing and identifying the feeling of *qi*.

It might seem that you can't open your hand as much the first way because you are wedded to the image of a balloon opening it, and a balloon is always convex. Actually, the image is only a way of identifying the feeling of a different way of using your muscles. Once that feeling is experienced—and it may take several tries before it is—you should put the image aside and work only from the feeling.

Experiment 2-3. Expanding and Releasing the Space between Your Fingers. Repeat the elements of the previous experiment, this time slightly opening the space between your fingers. Then allow the fingers to resume their natural, released spacing.

Experiment 2-4. Rotating Your Wrists. Stand with feet parallel. Extend one arm (say, your left arm) forward, in front of the body. Let the wrist find its neutral orientation (neither rotated to the right nor to the left). Next, rotate your palm downward in two different ways:

(a) The contractive way is to pull your left palm heel downward by contracting the muscles on the inside of your forearm and to pull your little finger upward by contracting the muscles on the outside of your forearm. This is the conventional way of moving by using contractive strength.

(b) The expansive way is to push your left palm heel downward by extending the muscles on the outside of your forearm and to push your left little finger upward by extending the muscles on the inside of your forearm. Notice that in this way of moving, the hand does not rotate fully, but in the first case it easily can. Also compare the amount of *qi* in your hand for the two ways.

Experiment 2-5. Extending Your Hamstrings. Stand with feet parallel. Lean forward and let your upper body hang from your hip joints, knees slightly bent. Relax your head, arms, and back as much as possible. Remaining so, next try lifting the pelvis in two different ways:

(a) The contractive way is to push the knees back, causing your legs to straighten. In this case, the muscles on the back of the legs are forced to lengthen by the contraction of muscles on the front of the legs. This is the conventional way of stretching

(continued on next page)

(b) The expansive way is to extend the legs by lifting the hip joints by extending the muscles on the back of the legs. These muscles lengthen by their own action rather than being forced to do so by contraction of the muscles on the front of the legs. Notice that in this way of moving, the legs do not totally straighten, but in the first case they easily can.

Experiment 2-6. Extending Your Hamstrings Again. Lie on your back on the floor, knees up. If you need to, place a pillow under your head to achieve an optimal alignment of your cervical vertebrae. After attaining the most-relaxed state you can, slowly lift one knee, balancing that leg on the pelvis, relaxing it as much as possible, and feeling the weight of your leg resting on the pelvis. Next, slowly extend the heel upward. Your working point is when you start to feel resistance. The goal now is to ease your heel upward without tensing the muscle on the front of your leg but by extending the muscles on the back of your leg. That is, the muscles that are getting longer are doing so at their own rate rather than being forced to do so by the opposing muscles. Should you start to feel the knee clench, you have substituted contractive movement for expansive strength.

Experiment 2-7. Extending Your Hip Adductors. First, watch a short video, available at the web address in the footnote below, of the author demonstrating this experiment.[7]

The hip adductors are muscles on the insides of your thighs that, when contracted, rotate your knees inward. Extending the adductors causes the knees to open outward.

Lie on your back on the floor, legs straight out, with heels touching each other. If you need to, place a pillow under your head to achieve an optimal alignment of the cervical vertebrae. Relaxing as much as possible, extend one knee horizontally a tiny amount away from the axis of your body. As you do so, rest the heel of that foot on the floor. Even if you have trouble at first, you should be able to eventually learn to move your knee an inch or more in this manner.

The conventional view of the above experiment is that contracting (shortening) muscles on the outside of the thigh is the only action that can cause the opposing hip adductors to lengthen. However, in the above action, the muscles on the insides of the leg are lengthening, but those on the outside are relaxed. If you feel the muscle on the inside of your left thigh with your hand, you will

---

7. https://www.chuckrowtaichi.com/AdductorExtension.mp4.

notice that it is activated when you move your knee outward by extension. If you feel (or have another person feel) the muscles on the outside and bottom of your left thigh, those muscles should be totally relaxed. These occurrences cannot be explained by the conventional view of muscular action.

Moreover, in doing this experiment, you should also be able to feel that your left hip joint is actually opening slightly. It is farfetched that there is a way for any of these actions to occur by contracting (shortening) muscles because contraction would compress rather than open that joint.

> **Experiment 2-8. Expanding Your Sphincter Muscles.** When you urinate or move your bowels, pay attention to what you do with your sphincter muscles, which are normally relaxed but taut. When you excrete, you extend these muscles and can directly feel that extension. Next, try contracting these same muscles. Note the difference in the feeling.

> **Experiment 2-9. Expanding Your Trachea.** Feel your trachea (windpipe) expand when you breathe in—and even more so when you yawn.

> **Experiment 2-10. Expanding Your Esophagus.** Next time you swallow supplements or other pills, notice how you expand your esophagus.

> **Experiment 2-11. Expanding Your Nostrils and Nasal Passages** Feel your nostrils flare and your nasal passages expand when you inhale. I have found this ability to be valuable in fully opening my nasal passages before falling asleep, thereby preventing mouth breathing.

> **Experiment 2-12. Extending Your Head Upward.** While standing in your best, relaxed posture, extend your head upward by creating subtle expansion of the space between the cervical vertebrae. The movement should be almost microscopic. How could extending the head upward be done by contracting muscles?

Experiment 2-13. Tilting Your Head Sideways. While standing in your best, relaxed posture, tilt your head two ways:

(a) The contractive way is to pull your head to the side by contracting the muscles on the side toward which your head is tilting. That way forces the muscles on the other side to lengthen.

(b) The expansive way is to extend the muscles on the side that is getting longer and just relax the muscles on the other side.

How to Confirm That You Are Using Expansive Strength

The question naturally arises: "I think I am using expansive strength, but how do I know if I am really doing so?" First, when doing Taiji movements, it is essential to release contractive strength so completely that every part of your body moves fluidly and responds to tiny amounts of momentum. Whereas being relaxed is necessary to attain *nei jin* (expansive strength), it is not sufficient. One test of the use of *nei jin* is that in practicing push-hands, your partner will be able to move you easily with a very small amount of force yet sense that all parts of your body are unified and your arms are expanded and potentially able to express a large amount of power without being stiff ("iron wrapped in cotton"). Another test is to assess the feeling of your muscles when you think that you are using expansive strength. Then try achieving that action by contracting muscles instead. You should feel a noticeable difference between the two types of strength, and that difference becomes even greater with practice. Namely, expansion involves a unified feeling of electrical stimulation, and contraction involves a sensation that is pronounced midway between the joints.

Experiment 2-14. Do the "Beginning" movement of the form. Start by standing for a period of time, attaining the deepest state of *song* possible. Feel the weight of everything, especially your arms. Relax your chest, shoulders, lower abdomen—everything. When you start raising your arms, the movement should be as slow and relaxed as possible. Feel how heavy your arms are and how hard it is to lift them. Perhaps you won't be able to get your wrists near shoulder level. That's because you have shed use of contractive strength. Next, extend your hands, not by pulling the fingers upward but by extending your palms. Then let your forearms lower by gravity rather than pulling your elbows back. As your arms continue to lower, extend the heels of your hands, again, rather than pulling your fingers upward.

(continued on next page)

When your hands reach their lowest position, note the swelling in them due to the increased hydraulic pressure. This effect is passive; that is, it doesn't result from your intention to create that pressure—just from the action of lowering your arms and the effect of gravity.

Now bend one elbow and bring that forearm to horizontal. Notice that the pressure and swelling subside. Without moving your arm, try to restore the feeling of pressure without any outward movement, using only your intention. If you are able to do so, then you have succeeded in achieving expansive strength.

Important: The "Beginning" movement is the prototype for lifting and lowering your arms in *all* movements of the form!

Experiment 2-15. Before leaving the prior experiment (Experiment 2-14), extend the expansion into your forearms, chest, and every other part of your body. Then intensify the level of expansion. At the same time, slowly experiment with different shapes of your arms. When you find a shape that maximizes the desired effect, capture that feeling so you can recreate it later.

A Promising Mechanism for Expansive Strength

Dr. Gerald Pollack has been directing research on hitherto disregarded properties of water and cellular phenomena at Washington State University for decades and has discovered an important feature based on the restructuring of water under certain conditions. Watch his video on some unusual aspects of water.[8]

Under the action of electricity, water can form a gel with properties of strength and extension. Because these properties are not similarly displayed by the commonly recognized phases of water, namely, liquid, solid, and gas, Pollack has called this state "the fourth phase of water." He has been able to shed light on a number of phenomena displayed by water that are otherwise unexplained.

Our cells and intracellular fluids are primarily water, and bioelectricity abounds in our bodies. Pollack's research suggests that our bioelectricity can restructure water in cells and tissues, resulting in their expansion.[9,10]

---

8. https://www.youtube.com/watch?v=i-T7tCMUDXU&feature=youtu.be.

9. Gerald H. Pollack, *Cells, Gels, and the Engines of Life* (Seattle, WA: Ebner and Sons Publishing, 2001).

10. Gerald H. Pollack, *The Fourth Phase of Water* (Seattle, WA: Ebner and Sons Publishing, 2013).

I have been pondering Dr. Pollack's research for the past several years. The concept that water in the cells can be made to expand and change in structure is quite satisfying because it closely matches what I experience with expansive strength; namely, I feel that I am sending electricity to my tissues, and it feels as though the water within is expanding as a consequence. In fact, before learning of Dr. Pollack's research, I experienced those effects for quite some time and described them as "hydraulic pressure."[11] Moreover, the writings of the Taiji Classics also utilize water analogies.

If the expansion of intra- and intercellular water can result from the application of bioelectricity, it nicely explains why expansive strength can be sustained without fatigue longer than for muscular contraction: aside from the chemical energy required for its neural activation, muscular contraction requires additional amounts of chemical energy from stores of glycogen. Then, muscular contraction results in the production of the irritating waste products and restricts the circulation of blood, which transports oxygen and nutrients into muscles and nerves and waste products out. Chemicals required for contraction soon become depleted, and irritating waste products build up. These factors limit the time that contraction can be sustained.

On the other hand, if expansion is based on an intrinsic property of water, it may only require bioelectricity for its activation—no chemical energy other than that for activation is needed, and no irritating waste products would be expected to result. In fact, a wonderful byproduct of expansion is that circulation of blood is not restricted but actually increased, and there is good reason to expect the accompanying bioelectricity to be therapeutic.

---

11. Robert Chuckrow, *Tai Chi Dynamics*, 8, 9, 19, 47.

Chapter 3
"Swimming on Land"

Professor Cheng's Advice

Cheng Man-ch'ing wrote about the importance of what is described as "swimming on land,"[1] "swimming in air,"[2] and "dry swimming."[3] We are advised in these writings to imagine the air as having the resistance and consistency of water when doing Taiji movement.

> Man lives on land. His long familiarity with air often makes him forget about its existence. Since it lacks solidity and shape, it eludes attention or easy mental grasp by the beginner. To liken air to water aids the imagination. It is like water in the sense that if one pretends to swim while out of water, his movements automatically conform to the principles of Taiji. By this practice, the novice will ultimately "feel" the air to be heavy in the sense that he feels water to be heavy. At this stage his body has become lighter and more pliable than that of the average man. This feeling of buoyancy and suppleness derives from firmly rooting the feet and using the body in "dry swimming." Functionally, this slow movement against an imagined resistance will ultimately create great speed in responding to a fighting situation.[4]

Professor Cheng considered "swimming on land" to be so important that he devoted a whole chapter to it in his *Thirteen Treatises*. In that chapter, Professor Cheng says:

> As you make progress the air will not only feel heavier than water, it will feel like iron.[5]

---

1. Cheng Man-ch'ing, *Cheng Tzu's Thirteen Treatises on T'ai Chi Ch'uan*, trans. Benjamin Pang Jen Lo and Martin Inn (Berkeley, CA: North Atlantic Books, 1981), 36–39.
2. Cheng Man-ch'ing and Robert W. Smith, *T'ai Chi: The "Supreme Ultimate" Exercise for Health, Sport, and Self Defense* (Rutland, VT: Charles E. Tuttle Co.,1967), 10.
3. Cheng Man-ch'ing, *Tai Chi Chuan: A Simplified Method of Calisthenics for Health and Self Defense*, North Atlantic (Berkeley, CA: North Atlantic Books, 1985), 12.
4. Cheng and Smith, *T'ai-Chi*, 10.
5. Cheng, *Cheng Tzu's Thirteen Treatises*, 39.

My Initial Skepticism

For a long time, I had difficulty in reconciling this concept with Professor Cheng's frequent admonitions to relax completely and surrender to gravity (*song*). I reasoned that using any muscular force against an imaginary resistance would also require generating a counter force by the opposing muscles and that pitting one muscle group against another would lock the body and prevent free movement. Such a condition also seems antithetical to the principle of non-action.

In addition, some classmates of mine who tried practicing against resistance appeared to be using a substantial amount of brute strength. I considered that way to be wrong and abstained from practicing swimming on land.

My Eventual Realization

I later saw that Professor Cheng used the words *imagination* and *imagined*. At no point did he suggest exerting any actual strength. Then I remembered that it is known that the mere thought of doing a physical action is accompanied by production of minute bioelectrical impulses that would ordinarily initiate that action. But such impulses are below the threshold for producing any outward exertion of strength. So imagining resistance need not involve pitting muscles against each other. Therefore, taking Professor Cheng's advice to mean imagining the air as having the resistance of water does not at all contradict his advice to relax.

More recently it occurred to me that when you relax completely (thereby subduing use of contractive strength) and imagine using strength, you are then more apt to produce the bioelectricity associated with expansive rather than contractive strength.

So imagining resistance can be thought of as an activity for training the bioelectrical system to stimulate expansive strength. Because doing so results in a perception of using strength without outwardly exerting it, it provides an effective feedback system for learning to achieve expansive strength and then increasing its intensity. That idea explains Professor Cheng's statement about the air feeling as though it has the resistance of iron.

It is evident that in promoting "swimming on land," Professor Cheng was revealing a tool for recognizing and then cultivating the internal state of strength called *nei jin* (internal strength), essential for both the health and self-defense aspects of Taiji. Cultivating such a state requires ferreting out and then relinquishing contractive muscular action.

As this new bioelectrical action becomes increasingly intense, more-widely distributed, and more under conscious volition, the movements are then increasingly done by using that kind of strength. Now there is a feeling of exertion but without any sensation that muscles are contracting. In my view, what you are feeling is the bioelectricity produced and its resulting expansion of the water in your tissues.

To see a truly impressive use of expansion in doing Taiji movement, please watch the first five minutes of this YouTube video of Wang Shu-chin (1904–1981).[6]

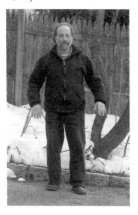

Fig. 3-1. The author standing in the "Beginning" Taiji posture, imagining water pushing his hands and arms from behind.

Experiment 3-1. On more than one occasion, one of my teachers, Harvey Sober, had us try this experiment: stand in a 50-50 stance, with feet parallel and shoulder-width apart ("Beginning" posture) (Figs. 3-1 and 3-2). Attain a state of *song*. Slowly rotate your elbows forward and out sideways. Then rotate your palms to face the rear. These three modifications should be independently fine-tuned experimentally to maximize the feeling of *qi* (swelling and tingling of the palms and forearms). Then imagine water coming from behind, pushing your hands forward. Imagine pushing back on the water without tensing muscles. You should feel the *qi* increase. After a while, the resistance will appear to be very great even though you are not tensing anything. If all goes well, you should now be in a state of expansion. Capture that expanded feeling and lock it in so you can recreate it later.

Next, try to intensify the expansion and spread it everywhere in your body. When you are in that expanded state, someone who tries to move your arm should not feel resistance resulting from contractive strength but, instead, feel that your arm is connected to every part of your body.

---

6. https://www.youtube.com/watch?v=JnhEwTAQr7Q&t=177s.

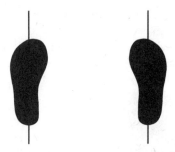

Fig. 3-2. The feet in a 50-50 stance, with the centerlines of the feet parallel. The feet are shoulder width apart, which means that the separation of the ankle joints equals that of the shoulder joints.

Experiment 3-2. If you succeed in achieving the state described in Experiment 3-1, now look at your hands, note their color and any swelling, and compare with their normal state.

The Mental Aspect

We previously quoted Prof Cheng's claim that practicing swimming on land "will ultimately create great speed in responding to a fighting situation." That claim is consistent with the heightened activity of bioelectrical readiness required for producing that state. As Sam Chin Fan-siong said, "The motor is running." In other words, you are alert and ready to go and don't need to insert the key and start the engine.

> The form is like that of a falcon about to seize a rabbit, and the *shen* (spirit) is like that of a cat about to catch a rat.[7]
>
> —Wu Yu-hsiang

"Zombie-Style Taiji"

Many Taiji practitioners work on and succeed in doing movements with the minimum strength. But because they were told not to use strength, they never attain expansive strength (*nei jin*). Instead, they are still using contractive strength (*li*), albeit minimally. That condition, sometimes called "floating," is lifeless and unconnected. Thus it is a sort of "zombie-style." Anyone who has

---

7. Benjamin Pang Jeng Lo, Martin Inn, Robert Amacker, and Susan Foe, eds., *The Essence of T'ai Chi Ch'uan* (Berkeley, CA: North Atlantic Books, 1985), 59.

cultivated expansive strength can instantly recognize the difference between use of *jin* and *li* in another person's movements.

When at Cheng's school, Shi Zhong, I noticed a student doing the form in a super-relaxed manner. Professor Cheng happened to walk by at that moment and said to him, "Too *yin*." I don't recall whether it was said directly in English by Professor Cheng or through a translator who was accompanying him.

Swimming on Land Is Only a Tool for Recognizing *Nei Jin*

It is important to understand that once the proper internal state is recognized and practiced, that state should then be recreated directly. At that point, imagining resistance is no longer necessary and should be set aside (see the section "Dangers of Overusing Images in Movement Arts" in Chapter 15).

The ultimate goal is to be able to spread bioelectrical activity throughout the whole body at will, expressing potential expansive strength in every direction with minimal muscular contraction.

Consider, for example, doing "Brush Knee," which is an early movement in various Taiji forms. A simplistic way of practicing "swimming on land" in that movement might be to imagine that the upper hand is striking and that the lower hand is circling the opponent's punching hand to his knee. Instead, I view imagining resistance to be just a tool for recognizing the skill of sending bioelectricity, resulting in expansion. When that skill is learned, one's intention can increase the breadth of that electrification. Eventually, the whole body feels like steel but still remains relaxed, pliable, and responsive. The feeling is one of having tremendous strength in every direction—not just in that of the movement. The resulting *qi* then permeates every part of the body with remarkable intensity.

Chapter 4

Elucidation of Famous Masters' Sayings on Mind, Qi, and Strength

This chapter will attempt to shed light on the various sayings and writings of famous Taiji masters concerning the relationships of mind, *qi*, and internal and external strength.

Li, Jin, and *Nei Jin*

In everyday Chinese speech, *li* and *jin* are used interchangeably for *strength* (see Fig. 4-1 for their characters). Also, Chinese-English dictionaries translate these words as having almost the same meaning. However, in martial arts, where specialized words are used, *li* refers to untrained physical strength, and *jin* implies a trained, sophisticated strength.

A further source for confusion is that martial *jin* can refer to *any* sophisticated strength, including that of hard styles. Technically, *nei jin* (*nei* means *internal*) is more appropriate to use for the expansive strength of Taiji and other internal styles. However, those who speak or write about Taiji often omit the adjective *nei*, and *jin* is simply used to mean *nei jin*.[1]

In English translations of the Taiji Classics to which we will next refer, the distinction between *li* and *jin* is sometimes unclear, and *jin* and *nei jin* are often used interchangeably. In what follows, the reader will need to keep in mind the above distinctions and pitfalls.

---

1. See http://www.ycgf.org/Articles/TJ_Jin/TJ_Jin1.html for a clear discussion of *jin*, *li*, and other specialized words.

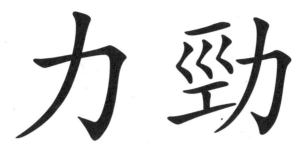

Fig. 4-1. The characters for *li* (left) and *jin* (right). In everyday discourse, *li* and *jin* are usually used interchangeably to mean strength. But when used in Taiji, *li* refers to untrained physical strength, and *jin* implies a trained, sophisticated strength.

Qi, Breath, and Internal and External Strength

Whereas Qigong has flourished as both a theory and as a practice for thousands of years, *qi* is still not adequately explained nor is its existence even accepted by Western science. But for anyone who has practiced Qigong or Neigong[2] sufficiently to experience *qi* and its healing effects, there is little need for science to affirm its validity. Nevertheless, in China and the United States there is currently ongoing scientific research into *qi* and the herbs of traditional Chinese medicine. Nevertheless, in China and the United States, there is currently ongoing scientific research into *qi* and the herbs of Traditional Chinese Medicine.

The Taiji Classics[3,4] frequently refer to the importance of understanding the relationships among *qi*, breath, and strength. Reading these old writings can be quite confusing—partly because they originated in old Chinese, then were translated into Modern Chinese, and were next translated into English. For example, *jin* and *li* are two frequently used Chinese words, each for a very different kind of strength. These words have no direct English counterparts, and some English translations use strength indiscriminately for both. Moreover, the word *qi* can be used for breath, a certain kind of strength, or even something not understood at that time. We now know about hydraulic pressure, and much about how bodily movement is initiated by the electrical effects of nerve impulses. Perhaps some of what the ancients called *qi* can now

---

2. Qigong involves movement to cultivate the flow of *qi*, and Neigong additionally involves intentionally creating an internal state that intensifies the *qi*.

3. Benjamin Pang Jeng Lo, Martin Inn, Robert Amacker, and Susan Foe, eds., *The Essence of T'ai Chi Ch'uan* (Berkeley, CA: North Atlantic Books, 1985).

4. Douglas Wile, comp. and trans., *T'ai Chi Touchstones: Yang Family Secret Transmissions* (Brooklyn, NY: Sweet Ch'i Press, 1983).

be interpreted in such terms,[5,6]and some English translations use strength indiscriminately for both. Moreover, the word qi can be used for breath, a certain kind of strength, or even something not understood at that time. Now we know about hydraulic pressure, and much about how bodily movement is initiated by the electrical effects of nerve impulses. Perhaps some of what the ancients called qi can now be interpreted in such terms."

But there are more reasons for confusion: in the past, Taijiquan was secret, and instructions were written to be understood by inner students but not outsiders. Also, knowledge common to the modern world was not then part of the Chinese conceptual framework and was unknown to the old Taiji masters. Such knowledge includes (a) the scientific and precise manner of explaining bodily states, forces, and movement; (b) the difference between conscious and subconscious thought; and (c) the manner in which cause and effect is scientifically determined. Even now, with all that's known, cause and effect is incorrectly asserted in some studies purporting to be scientific.

In order to understand the ancient writings so that the many current Taiji practitioners can maximize its wonderful health and self-development benefits, we need to use creative skills, an open mind, and modern tools such as the concepts of science (hydraulic pressure, wave motion, momentum, gravity, effects of bodily electricity, etc.).

Consider the following English translation of "Expositions of Insights into the Practice of the Thirteen Postures" by Wu Yu-hsiang:

> The *xin* (mind) mobilizes the *qi* (breath). Make the *qi* sink calmly; then it gathers and permeates the bones. The *qi* mobilizes the body. Make it move smoothly, then it easily follows (the direction of) the *xin*.
>
> The *xin* (mind) is the commander, the *qi* (breath) the flag, and the waist is the banner. The waist is like an axle and the *qi* is like the wheel.[7]

—Wu Yu-hsiang

5. Lo et al., *The Essence of T'ai Chi Ch'uan.*
6. Wile, *T'ai Chi Touchstones.*
7. Lo et al., *The Essence of T'ai Chi Ch'uan,* 43 and 44, respectively.

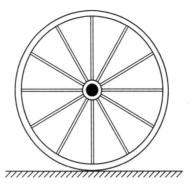

Fig. 4-2. A spoked wheel. As the wheel rolls, the lowest spoke exerts an upward support on the axle and an outward force on the rim. The other spokes keep the wheel from changing shape. In a modern pneumatic wheel, the air pressure supplies the expansive support.

The idea here is that the mind is the agent that mobilizes *qi*. The *qi*, in turn, then mobilizes the body under the action of the mind. An axle without a wheel can't do much. But how can the *qi* be like a wheel? Clearly, the wheel (Fig. 4-2) provides and "mobilizes" outward (expansive) strength that does not collapse under external pressure. So the question is, how can *qi* be related to such strength?

Consider the following English translation of an explanation by Yang Cheng-fu.

The Meaning of Strength Versus *Qi* in *Taiji*

Qi runs through the channels of the internal membranes and sinews.[8] Strength issues from the blood, flesh, skin, and bones. Thus, those possessed of strength are externally sturdy in their skin and bones, that is, in their physical form; those possessed of *qi* have internal strength in their sinews, that is, their charisma (*hsiang*). *Qi* and blood work to strengthen the internal; the *qi* of the blood works to strengthen the external.

In summary, if you understand the function of the two words—*qi* and *blood*—then you will naturally know the origin of strength and *qi*. If you know the nature of strength and *qi*, you will know the difference between using strength and mobilizing *qi*. Mobilizing *qi* in the sinews and using strength in the skin and bones are two vastly different things.[9]

When Yang talks about the difference between strength and *qi*, the strength he is referring to is apparently *li*—not *jin*. And the implication is that *qi* is the desired kind of strength (*jin*).

---

8. Medically, *sinew* is a synonym for *tendon*. But older meanings pertain to strength or nerve energy.

9. Wile, *T'ai Chi Touchstones*, 86.

The relationship between *qi* and *jin* is immediately felt when doing Neigong (literally translated as *internal skill*, which involves intentionally opening the body to free up pathways of *qi*),[10] exemplified by the Jade Belt (Fig. 4-3).[11] When you practice the Jade Belt, the arms (and all other parts of the body) are expanded outward by intention, which initiates relaxed but expansive power. After only a few minutes, the entire body becomes filled with *qi* and a feeling of expanded strength. So when our bioelectricity is directed by our intention to activate the tissues to produce expansive strength, that is when the *qi* is experienced the most. It therefore makes sense that expansive strength and *qi* are interconnected.

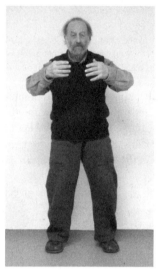

Fig. 4-3. The author in a 50-50 variation of the Jade-Belt stance.

It is not unreasonable that the ancient masters' idea that *qi* is a kind of strength stems from the strong interrelationship of *qi* and expansive strength.

---

10. *Neigong* means *internal skill or work*. Neigong is similar to Qigong except that Neigong involves actively using the mind to create the conditions for maximizing the flow of *qi* by opening the body and, thereby, the channels of *qi* flow.

11. See variations of the Jade Belt at the eight-minute point in the author's youtube.com video: https://www.youtube.com/watch?v=bAhNA23UTeE&t=8s.

An Analysis of Cheng Man-ch'ing's Distinction between Two Different Types of Strength

The excerpt below was written by Cheng Man-ch'ing. Note that the quoted text is an English translation of Professor Cheng's original book, which was written in Chinese. Bear in mind that to properly translate such a difficult subject, the translator not only needs to be fluent in Chinese and English but also adept at the subject discussed.

> When the body is entirely emptied of force, a "tenacious strength" will develop from the foot. Tenacious strength may be distinguished from force in that the former has root in the foot while the latter has not. When in action, tenacity may be likened to a strong vine which is pliable, and force to a stick which is rigid. Hence we say: "tenacity is alive, force is inert." Tenacity is the resilience or tonicity of living muscles however relaxed they may be. The muscles being relaxed, tenacity cannot involve the bones. Force, on the other hand, is derived from binding the bones together into a wooden (rigid) system. Tradition has handed down, as a secret formula, that "tenacity is derived from muscle; force, from bones."[12]

Next, the above paragraph is rewritten below, with the word *force* replaced by the words *contractive strength* and *tenacity* and *tenacious strength* replaced by the words *expansion* and *expansive strength*, respectively. Please read the following rephrased paragraph, and compare with the content of Chapters 2 and 3:

> When the body is entirely emptied of contractive strength, a "tenacious strength" (expansive strength) will develop from the foot. Expansive strength may be distinguished from contractive strength in that the former has root in the foot while the latter has not. When in action, expansive strength may be likened to a strong vine which is pliable, and contractive strength to a stick which is rigid. Hence we say: "Expansive strength is alive, contractive strength is inert." Expansive strength is the resilience or tonicity of living muscles however relaxed they may be. The muscles being relaxed, expansive strength cannot involve the bones. Contractive strength, on the other hand, is derived from binding the bones together into a wooden (rigid) system. Tradition has handed down, as a secret formula, that "expansive strength is derived from muscle; contractive strength, from bones."

---

12. Cheng Man-ch'ing, *T'ai Chi Chuan: A Simplified Method of Calisthenics for Health & Self-Defense* (Richmond, VA: North Atlantic Books, 1981), 16–17.

An Attempt to Further Elucidate What Professor Cheng Wrote

As you release contractive tension, there is a feeling that the whole body becomes liquefied. Then, as you shift and sink into a foot during a transition, it feels like the liquid in your body is thereby pressurized and expands everywhere, especially into your arms (imagine squeezing the base of a tube of toothpaste and how the nozzle end expands). However, it helps to additionally send the right bioelectricity to enhance the expansive effect. That's where reverse breathing can be an important tool. Reverse breathing involves expansion, which sympathetically produces an expansive effect throughout the body.[13] Once that effect is recognized and practiced, it can be done independently of any particular way of matching breathing with movements.

Whereas any movement can be utilized for working on expansion, the very first movement ("Preparation") is an especially good one. As I release and sink into my right foot, I use my intention to correspondingly pressurize the liquid in my arms, causing them to expand slightly outward from my body. As I turn to the right, I use that expansion to rotate my arms so the palms face the rear. The "Preparation" movement symbolizes the separation of *yin* and *yang*. Sinking into the right foot causes it to be *yin* (yielding, supportive, earthy). The result is the production of *yang* in the arms and left leg (active, expansive, upward, outward).

Both expansion and contraction involve bioelectrical action, so initially it is hard to distinguish between those two types of strength. So if you are in doubt as to whether or not you are actually expanding instead of contracting, it is possible to check by then contracting the muscles in your arms and feeling the difference, which should be quite noticeable.

Everyone can produce expansive strength—it's mainly a matter of recognizing how to do it. Try yawning intensely, and feel the effect throughout your body. Try expanding your midsection to its front, sides, and rear. Once you recognize the feeling, then recreate and practice doing it increasingly fully and intensely, working up slowly, over time.

Professor Cheng's advice about imagining the air to have the resistance of water, discussed in Chapter 3, is another tool for recognizing expansive strength.

13. Robert Chuckrow, *Tai Chi Dynamics* (Wolfeboro, NH: YMAA Publication Center, 2008): 13–23.

An Analysis of Yang Cheng-fu's Commentary on Strength

The following is the translation of an oral transmission by Yang Cheng-fu. It is the sixth of Yang Cheng-fu's ten important points for Taijiquan, dictated to one of his senior students, Chen Wei-ming, who wrote it down and published it. It is included in *The Essence of T'ai Chi Ch'uan: The Literary Tradition*.[14]

Use Mind and Not Force

The Taijiquan Classics say, "all of this means use *yi* (mind) and not *li* (force)." In practicing Taijiquan, the whole body relaxes. Don't let one ounce of force remain in the blood vessels, bones and ligaments to tie yourself up. Then you can be agile and able to change. You will be able to turn freely and easily. Doubting this (not using *li*), how can you increase your power?

The body has meridians like the ground has ditches and trenches. If not obstructed, the water can flow. If the meridian is not closed, the *qi* (breath) goes through. If the whole body has hard force and it fills up the meridians, the *qi* and blood stop and the turning is not smooth and agile. Just pull one hair and the whole body is off-balance. If you use *yi* not *li*, then the *yi* goes to a place (in the body) and the *qi* follows it. The *qi* and the blood circulate. If you do this every day and never stop, after a long time you will have *nei jin* (real internal force). The Taijiquan Classics say, "when you are extremely soft, then you become extremely hard and strong." Someone who has extremely good Taijiquan gongfu has arms like iron wrapped with cotton, and the weight is very heavy. As for those who practice the external schools, when they use *li*, they reveal *li*. When they don't use *li*, then they are too light and floating. Their *jin* (internal force) is external and locked together. The *li* of the external schools is easily led and moved and not to be esteemed.[15]

—Yang Cheng-fu

Interpretation of "Use *I* (Mind) and Not *Li* (Force).

We cannot interpret that *yi* transmits an *illusion* of strength to others because the Classics say that the arms become like iron. If anything, the strength is actual and physical and is described by Yang Cheng-fu as "concealed." However, the strength referred to is different from *li* (ordinary strength) and is often called *nei jin*, which is "sophisticated," internal strength.

Thus, the mind is causing something to happen in the body that does not occur normally and, therefore, must be recognized and cultivated. That is, the everyday strength we exert requires no specialized training or unusual action of

---

14. Lo et al., *The Essence of T'ai Chi Ch'uan*, 87.
15. Lo et al., *The Essence of T'ai Chi Ch'uan*, 87.

the mind—just our desire to exert it. So the cultivation of *nei jin* (internal strength) needs special training and use of the conscious mind (*yi*).

The accepted way that the mind can generate physical strength is by means of electricity traveling from the brain and spinal cord, along the nerves, to the tissues. For *nei jin*, the electrical impulses involved are evidently not of a nature to cause muscles to contract but something else. We are told to relax completely in order to shed the use of contractive strength. Such emptying is necessary for learning to generate strength through the expansion, initiated by *yi*, thereby consciously sending bioelectricity that results in a kind of strength that is different from contraction.

Our interpretation here is that the strength referred to is expansive. It is understandable that the use of contractive strength would mask recognition of the difference between the two types of strength. Cultivating expansive strength requires long, consistent practice to develop because it is unfamiliar, whereas contractive strength is familiar and habitual.

The *qi* flow is then enhanced by the bioelectrical stimulation to the tissues and freed by the release of contractive tension that blocks it. So it makes sense that the ancient Taiji masters, who were not trained in Western physiology and may not have understood the role of bioelectricity, would identify the state of expansion with increased *qi* and think that *qi* is *responsible* for the resulting strength. Instead, it is likely the other way around; namely, the *qi* is a result not a cause. Reversing cause and effect is not uncommon for those untrained in science and even for some that are so trained.

Next, the above paragraph is rewritten below, with the word *force* replaced by the words *contractive strength* and the word *mind* replaced by the words *expansive strength*. After all, ordinary strength develops automatically, but expansive strength requires mindful cultivation. Now, please read a rephrasing of the prior quote of Yang Cheng-fu, and compare with what I have been saying about expansive strength in prior chapters.

Use the Mind and Not Contractive Strength

The Taijiquan Classics say, "all of this means use expansive strength and not contractive strength." In practicing Taijiquan the whole body relaxes. Don't let one ounce of contractive strength remain in the blood vessels, bones, and ligaments to tie yourself up. Then you can be agile and able to change. You will be able to turn freely and easily. Doubting this (not using contractive strength), how can you increase your power?

The body has meridians like the ground has ditches and trenches. If not obstructed, the water can flow. If the meridian is not closed, the *qi* (breath) goes through. If the whole body has hard force and it fills up the meridians, the *qi* and blood stop and the turning is not smooth and agile. Just pull one hair and the whole body is off-balance. If you use expansive strength not contractive strength, then the expansive strength goes to a place (in the body) and the *qi* follows it. The *qi* and the blood circulate. If you do this every day and never stop, after a long time you will have *nei jin* (real internal force). The Taijiquan Classics say, "when you are extremely soft, then you become extremely hard and strong." Someone who has extremely good Taijiquan gongfu has arms like iron wrapped with cotton, and the weight is very heavy. As for those who practice the external schools, when they use contractive strength, they reveal contractive strength. When they don't use contractive strength, then they are too light and floating. Their *jin* (trained force) is external and locked together The contractive strength of the external schools is easily led and moved and not to be esteemed.[16]

It is interesting that a description of the state experienced is somehow related to the image of blood or water flowing. That idea is consistent with our hypothesis that expansive strength is related to a change of state of water in bodily tissues.

Breath and the *Dan Tian*

The *dan tian* is a region centered an inch below the navel and about one-third of the way from front to back. It is a part of the anatomy that is unrecognized by Western science. The Chinese, on the other hand view it as the body center, both anatomically and as a region for the accumulation of *qi*. It is also an important acupuncture point. The Japanese also recognize the importance of the *dan tian* and refer to it as *hara*. In Japan, some people wear scarves called *hara maki* around their lower abdomens to nurture their *qi*, or as they call it, *ki*.

Many practitioners lament that they do not feel the *dan tian*, perhaps because during form practice, they are doing shallow, natural breathing. Such breathing just doesn't sufficiently activate that region.

When contractive strength is sufficiently released, the body liquefies, resulting in a hydraulic-pressure gradient. That is, the lower in the body, the greater the pressure. The greatest pressure in the trunk of the body is in the lower abdomen, which contributes to a sensation of activation of that region.

During the inhalation in natural breathing, the lower abdomen expands and pressurizes. In reverse breathing, such pressure occurs continually, increasing and decreasing but not totally releasing. The effects of breathing can be felt as a swelling of the region having the description of the *dan tian*.

---

16. Here is an example of how the word *jin* is interpreted as internal strength or force, but actually *jin* is any kind of refined strength, including external strength (*wei jin*), which is what Yang Cheng-fu evidently meant. More precisely, *nei jin* is internal force.

Health Aspects

Think of the benefits of *song kai*: (a) letting go of muscular contraction promotes free flow of blood, lymph, and *qi*; (b) the bioelectricity to the relaxed cells plus condensing and expanding the cells helps them expel metabolic waste and other impurities and to absorb oxygen and nutrients; (c) the nervous system is activated and finely trained by the rich neurological dialogue involved.

> Think over carefully what the final purpose is: to lengthen life and maintain youth.[17]

—Unknown Author

Martial Aspects

Using contractive strength to exert an outward force on the other person means that muscles are pulling bones (tension). By contrast, use of expansive strength means that hydraulic pressure (expansion) is producing an outward force on the other person. The following two examples illustrate how use of expansion in push-hands practice or in a self-defense situation can produce a substantial advantage:

1. Because contractive strength is used by almost everyone in almost every situation, it is quite familiar and can easily be "read" by another person to know your intention. By contrast, expansive strength is unconventional, hidden, hard to interpret, and therefore deceptive.

When you exert contractive force on an opponent, say to deflect his incoming arm, he immediately reads the tension involved, recognizes your intention, is alerted, and acts to increase his force to prevent you from deflecting him. This initiates a succession of escalations of force by each person in turn. So a fight ensues, and the stronger person wins. But what if you are not as strong as your opponent or are old, injured, or sick? Then you will lose.

Instead, if you use expansive force, the opponent feels as though he contacted your body, which then turns. He is not alerted but instead perceives that his action caused your body to turn. He does not feel any reason to escalate his force and does not do so. As a consequence, he overextends, loses his balance, and is then easily controlled. For such an action, you don't need much expansive strength—only a few ounces.

The above example illustrates:

> The whole body is a hand
> and a hand is not a hand.[18]

—Cheng Man-ch'ing

---

17. Cheng Man-ch'ing, *Tai Chi Chuan*, 16–17.
18. Lo et al., *The Essence of T'ai Chi Ch'uan*, 95.

Professor Cheng is saying here that all parts of the body must be unified, with no part moving or exerting strength independently.

2. Whether you exert contractive or expansive force on another person, the reaction to your force on him is an equal-and-opposite force, exerted backward on your body. This backward force is balanced by a forward force on your feet by the frictional force of the floor. Moreover, your legs must act in such a way as to push your feet into the floor and push your pelvis forward.

Now consider what happens when you use contraction to exert a force on another person. If he then adjusts in such a way as to lessen the force exerted on him, in order for you to maintain balance, you must immediately change the conditions of contractive tension of your legs, which are pushing the floor backward and your pelvis forward. Unless you lessen the contractive tension of your legs in exact accordance with his change (extremely difficult to do quickly), your legs push your body forward, causing you to momentarily lose your balance. Thus, each time you use contraction to exert a force on someone, you are dependent for your balance on what he does and on the time it takes you to recognize and process that change and adjust complex forces accordingly. An experienced practitioner can take advantage of even your slightest momentary imbalance—especially when he is initiating it.

By contrast, when you exert expansive force on another person, the forces within your body result from the hydraulic pressure of water within your body. Pascal's principle states that any change in the pressure at any point of a liquid causes exactly the same change at every other point in the liquid. Thus, if the person on whom you are exerting expansive force moves in such a way as to lessen the force exerted on him, that automatically results in an immediate reduction in hydraulic pressure throughout your body—all the way down your legs, to your feet. As a consequence, your arm may momentarily move forward but not your body. You don't lose your balance, and no processing or adjustment of the legs is required.

> The [nei] jin of the (whole) body, through practice becomes one unit . . . One must completely raise the spirit (pay attention) at the moment when the opponent's jin is just about to manifest but has not yet been released. My jin has already met his (jin), not late, not early. It is like using a leather (tinder) to light a fire, or like a fountain gushing forth.[19]

—Li I-yu

Note: The words within parentheses in the above quotation are the translator's, and the words within the square brackets are this author's. Also, note the analogy involving water.

---

19. Lo et al., *The Essence of T'ai Chi Ch'uan*, 76.

Mind, Breath, *Qi*, and Strength

Breath

Breathing is emphasized in many Taiji writings and by many Taiji teachers, not just for its oxygenating value but as a way of increasing *qi* and internal strength. Because a person takes millions of breaths per year, the expansive aspect of breathing—especially of reverse breathing—helps recognition of the mechanism for achieving expansive rather than contractive strength and spreading expansive action throughout the entire body.

Breathing, *qi*, and internal strength are all considered to be importantly connected, as indicated by the classical writings and by what my Taiji teachers have emphasized. Actually, Professor Cheng did not to my knowledge talk about breathing other than to say, "As the arms rise in the 'Beginning' movement, you are breathing in. The rest takes care of itself."

Knowing what I now do, I can see why Professor Cheng didn't talk more about breathing:

1. He didn't know English, so he had no idea of how his instruction and his answers to questions in Chinese were interpreted into English.
2. He knew how complicated the subject of breathing was and how problems could occur from an incorrect understanding. So it makes sense that he would avoid the subject. However, a knowledge of the mechanics of breathing and how it relates to *qi* and strength are extremely valuable.
3. From what I heard Professor Cheng say and from conversations with senior classmates, it seems that he did not approve of purposely matching breathing with movements.

In natural breathing, the lower abdomen expands and releases. In reverse breathing, the lower abdomen is in a subtle state of expansion that increases and decreases but does not release completely. Because the expansive nature of both natural and reverse breathing is so fundamental, breathing—especially reverse breathing—furthers expansion in other parts of the body. Thus, breathing is a precursor to expansive strength.

Expansive Strength

The nature of expansive strength is the release of contractive tension through-out the body, which enhances the flow of blood, lymph, and *qi*. Next, the amplification of bioelectricity that produces the expansion has a highly stimulating effect on the *qi*. Of course, for the electricity to be so guided into expansion rather than contraction, the mind must be engaged. So the connection between mind, breath, *qi* and strength makes sense. Of course, the ancients did not have the knowledge of physiological and neurological science to explain such a relationship other than to say the mind moves the *qi* and the *qi* moves the body. Or "use Mind, not strength."

The following passage is attributed to Yang Banhou:

> Power comes from the sinews. Strength comes from the bones. Looking at it purely physically, one who has great strength is able to carry many hundreds of pounds, but this is an externally showy action of bones and joints, a stiff strength. If on the other hand the power of your whole body is used, it may appear you are unable to lift hardly any weight at all, yet there is an internal robustness of essence and energy, and once you have achieved skill, you will seem to have something more wonderful than one who has the stiff sort of strength. Thus runs the method of physical training for self-cultivation.[20]

—Attributed to Yang Banhou [circa 1875]

Summary

Taiji teachers almost universally tell students to relax (*song*). The main reason for attaining *song* is to learn to recognize and weed out the use of contractive strength (*li*) so that when students are ready, they will be able to learn to generate and then use expansive strength (*nei jin*). This way of teaching is in accordance with the Taoist (Daoist) view, expressed by the saying, "An empty cup holds the most." Unfortunately, *nei jin* is very difficult for teachers to explain and consequently for students to recognize and manifest. Thus, many practitioners erroneously believe that any development of strength and its use in Taiji is wrong. Of course, a practitioner who lacks the ability to manifest expansive strength must use contractive strength but keep it to an absolute minimum, which results in limp, substanceless, floating, lifeless movement. As expansive strength is recognized and cultivated, *qi* is intensified and the Taiji movements become more continuous, circular, tension-free, and imbued with potential power.

---

20. Paul Brennan trans., *Taiji's Substance & Application*, Sept. 2013, https://brennantranslation. wordpress.com/2013/09/14/explaining-taiji-principles-taiji-fa-shuo/?fbclid=IwAR1H UgWy-U2ekQb0u-gtYY7T6p_5JLG37-31hee53d84nBLzo7dC_i3LqCc.

Chapter 5

Advantages of Expansion over Contraction in Taiji

Much of the analysis of this chapter is an amplification of parts of my book, *Tai Chi Dynamics*.[1]

Briskness of Regulation of Strength Compared for Both Types of Strength

Use of Contractive Strength

When contractive muscular strength is employed, nerve impulses from the brain and spinal cord cause muscle units to contract. The contracting muscles pull bones by means of their associated tendons, thereby producing external force and movement. When external conditions require a change in the contraction produced, that change requires a succession of events to occur: 1) Afferent nerve impulses arising from sensory stimuli (sense data) are transmitted to the central nervous system and brain for analysis. 2) The analytical part of the brain then perceives the need to regulate external force and movement in accordance with what is perceived. 3) Based on the perceived need, the analytical mind then generates a course of action. 4) Efferent (motor) neural impulses are then sent to muscles, causing force and movement for the required change. The time taken for this succession of neurological events can be long compared to the time in which external conditions can change, especially in a self-protection situation.

---

1. Robert Chuckrow, *Tai Chi Dynamics* (Wolfeboro, NH: YMAA Publication Center, 2008), 47–54.

Use of Expansive Strength

When you achieve a deep state of *song*, allowing the body to liquefy, contractive strength is then incompatible with that state and thereby minimized. So when strength is required while sustaining this liquefied state, instead of nerve impulses that are normally generated to cause muscles to contract, now bioelectricity is generated to expand and, thereby, pressurize and change the state of the water in the muscle cells and possibly other tissues.[2] This pressure extends to every relaxed region of the body. A principle in physics, mentioned earlier, called Pascal's principle, states:

> Any change in the pressure at any point in a confined liquid is accompanied by the same change in pressure at every other point.

During the exertion of external force, if any increase or decrease is required by external conditions, there is no need for any neurological activity or analytical processing. Because of Pascal's principle, as soon as there is a sudden increase or decrease in external force, the hydraulic pressure within the body automatically adjusts, virtually instantaneously.

Stability

One important distinction between contractive and expansive strength applies to the exertion of force on you by an opponent (or vice versa). A basic principle in physics that governs situations involving the application of force of one body on another is Newton's third law, which states:

> If object *A* exerts a force on object *B*, then *B* exerts an equal-and-opposite force on *A*.

This law applies to all bodies—sentient or not, stationary or moving. A corollary of Newton's third law is that it is impossible for you to exert a force on another person or object without that person or object exerting the same force back on you. It is a consequence of Newton's third law that, when a person exerts a force, say on a door, the door exerts an equal-and-opposite force on the person (the reaction) (see Fig. 5-1). This result holds whether the door moves or not![3]

---

2. The possibility exists that bioelectrical impulses beyond those from nerves are involved.

3. Not all equal-and-opposite forces are action/reaction. For example, equal-and-opposite forces that are on the same object are never action/reaction—as in the case of the downward force of gravity and the upward force of the floor on a stationary person.

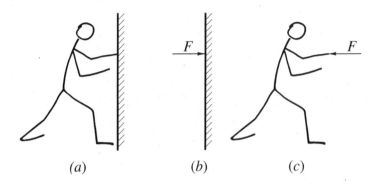

Fig. 5-1. (a) A person is pushing a door with a force of magnitude F to the right. (b) The force exerted by the person on the door. (c) The reaction force of an equal magnitude F to the left, exerted by the door on the person.

Thus, if someone exerts force on your body with his hand, your body automatically exerts a force back on his hand that is exactly equal in magnitude and opposite in direction to the force his hand exerts on your body. Similarly, when you place your hand on someone's body, now two forces come into play. One is the force that you are exerting on his body with your hand. The other is the equal-and-opposite force exerted on your hand by his body.

Neutralization

In Taiji, Newton's third law comes into play in causing an opponent to lose his balance (called "breaking the opponent's root") as follows: if an opponent A exerts a force F on me, according to Newton's third law, I automatically exert the same force F on A in the opposite direction (the reaction to A's force). In order to remain in balance, A must arrange things so that the total frictional force of the floor on his feet exerts a force that is opposite to the force I am exerting on him. If either of these two forces on A is removed or changed, A's balance will be disrupted until he readjusts the forces on himself (see Fig. 5-2 for the forces involved).

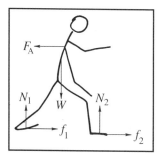

Fig. 5-2. All of the forces on person A when pushing person B are shown and labeled: F_A is the force on A, which is equal and opposite to the force that A exerts on B (the reaction to A's force on B). W is the weight of A (the gravitational force exerted by the earth on A's center of mass). N_1 is the upward force the floor exerts on A's rear foot, and N_2 is the upward force that the floor exerts on A's forward foot. Note that the sum of N_1 and N_2 is a force equal and opposite to W (A is balanced in the vertical direction). The force f_1 is the frictional force that the floor exerts on A's rear foot, and f_2 is the frictional force that the floor exerts on A's forward foot. Note that the sum of f_1 and f_2 is a force equal and opposite to F_A (A is balanced in the horizontal direction).

Assume that A exerts a force on me. Because I have control over the intensity of my reaction force on A, I can regulate and then suddenly release that force, causing F_A to momentarily go to zero. In order to restore balance in the horizontal direction, A must promptly reduce the frictional forces of the floor on his feet, pushing him forward. That restoration of balance requires a prompt reduction of the force of A's feet pushing backward on the floor. If A is using contractive strength, then A must perceive that change and make an adjustment. The time A takes to recover his loss of balance is then long enough for me to take advantage of it. However, if A is using expansive strength to exert force on me, then the hydraulic pressure everywhere within every part of A's body automatically releases almost instantaneously, with no conscious adjustment required. Such an immediate recovery prevents my taking advantage of any imbalance that A would otherwise have.

Experiment 5-1. The purpose of this experiment is to recognize the difference between contractive and expansive strength. Two students pair off in a harmonious stance (Fig. 5-3). One student A (on the left) assumes the posture "Ward Off," and the other student B (on the right) assumes "Push."

It is important for both partners to relax as much as possible and use a very small amount of strength. The person in "Ward Off" is the one actively pushing, and B supplies only the minimum pressure that prevents her hands from being moved backward. That is, the amount force is totally up to A.

If *A* uses contractive strength and *B* suddenly lets up, *A* will lose balance and her body will momentarily lurch forward. Instead, if *A* uses expansive strength and *B* suddenly lets up, *A* will not lose her balance or lurch forward—only her arm will move forward.

Moreover, when *A* uses contractive strength, *B* will feel that *A*'s strength originates in her upper body. But when *A* uses expansive strength, *B* will feel that *A*'s strength originates from the ground.

In doing this experiment, is important for both participants to share with each other what they experience.

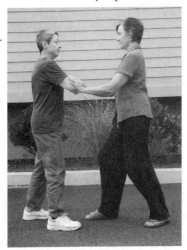

Fig. 5-3. Two students comparing the adaptive value of using expansive strength with that of using contractive strength.[4]

Alertness

In a state of expansion, the nervous system is highly activated. There is an alertness that provides an almost instantaneous response to any external change that requires it.

> The form is like that of a falcon about to seize a rabbit, and the *shen* (spirit) is like that of a cat about to catch a rat.[5]

—Wu Yu-hsiang

4. This photo was reproduced from Robert Chuckrow, *Tai Chi Dynamics* (Wolfeboro, NH: YMAA Publication Center, 2008), 49.

5. Benjamin Pang Jeng Lo, Martin Inn, Robert Amacker, and Susan Foe, eds., *The Essence of T'ai Chi Ch'uan, The Literary Tradition* (Berkeley, CA: North Atlantic Books, 1985), 59.

Endurance and Health Benefits

During the time that muscles are in a state of contraction, the flow of blood and *qi* are reduced, and cellular movement is restricted. These factors reduce (a) the cellular absorption of oxygen and nutrients and the removal of metabolic waste, (b) the ability for the cells to distribute their contents optimally, and (c) the amount of time that muscles can remain in a state of contraction without tiring.

By comparison, expansion does not result in such undesirable effects and can, therefore, be sustained longer. If expansion is based on an intrinsic property of water, as hypothesized in Chapter 2, then the use of chemical energy for contraction would not be required, thus additionally lengthening the time for sustaining expansion.

The cellular stimulation resulting from use of expansive strength also adds important health benefits beyond those of simply relaxing muscles. The bioelectricity that produces expansion actually *increases* the circulation of blood and *qi*. This increase can be felt and can even be visible as a substantial increase in coloration in one's extremities.

I have written about the idea that *qi* is very closely related to bioelectrical stimulation of cells, which causes beneficial micro-movement of them and assists in their absorption of oxygen and nutrients and elimination of wastes.[6] If the idea that *qi* is related to cellular stimulation by bioelectricity is correct, then increasing such stimulation in the absence of muscular contraction would explain an increase in *qi*.

Leverage and Fine-Motor Control

Three Classes of Levers

The lever is a rigid rod, straight or bent, that can rotate about a fixed point called *a fulcrum*. Force is applied to one point of the lever (the input), and force is exerted by another point (the output). Levers multiply force and reduce motion—or vice versa, depending on their design and use.

It should be noted that the rod can have any shape—it need not be a straight line—as long as it is resilient and does not distort under the stress of its action. Also, a combination of levers can be arranged so that the output of one can act on the input end of the next. Such a combination of levers is called a *compound lever*.

6. Robert Chuckrow, "A Biological Interpretation of Ch'i," *Qi: The Journal of Traditional Eastern Health & Fitness,* 21, no. 3 (Autumn, 2011).

The three classes of levers are described below.

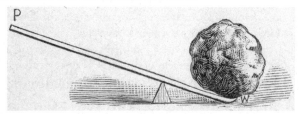

Fig. 5-4. A familiar (class-one) lever that multiplies applied force and reduces motion.[7]

The lever shown in Figure 5-4 is the most familiar version. Here, force (applied downward) at point P is multiplied by the ratio of the distance of P to the fulcrum Q divided by the distance of the fulcrum to the weight W being lifted. If that ratio were 2:1, the applied force required would be only half the weight of the stone, but the movement at P would be twice that of the weight (halving your force requires doubling your movement). The movement of the stone would be half that at P.

The lever shown in Figure 5-5 is also familiar. Here the fulcrum is at one end of the lever, and the input force is applied at the other end.

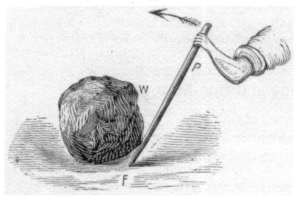

Fig. 5-5. A class-two lever that multiplies applied force and reduces motion.[8]

---

7. This figure was reproduced from Edward R. Shaw, *Physics by Experiment* (New York: Maynard, Merrill, & Co., 1897), 16.

8. This figure was reproduced from Edward R. Shaw, *Physics by Experiment*, 28

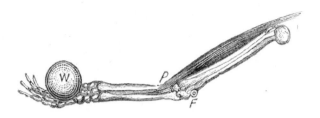

Fig. 5-6. A less-familiar (class-three) lever that multiplies motion and reduces force. *P* is the point of attachment of the biceps tendon to the radius bone of the forearm, and the elbow *F* is the fulcrum.[9]

In Figure 5-6, which shows an arm lifting a weight, the biceps tendon applies a force at *P*, and the fulcrum *F* is at the elbow. In this case, the force-and-motion-multiplying situation is reversed from that in Figures 5-4 and 5-5; namely, the motion of the weight is much greater than that of the applied force, and the applied force is much greater than the weight being lifted. This compromise between strength and mobility evidently has evolved based on its survival value for our ancestors and on the maximum strength and range of movement of muscular contractive motor units (sarcomeres).[10]

Fine-Motor Control

The result of the above physiological relationship between arm strength and motion is that the motion of the biceps is small and that of the weight is large. This relationship results in a lack of fine motor control when strength from muscular contraction is utilized. However, when expansive strength is applied, no such lack of control occurs.

Developing Bodily Unification

A major goal in Taiji movement is for all parts of the body to be interconnected and coordinate with each other as they move. Such unification is almost automatic when expansion is achieved and essentially impossible when it is not.

> Remember, when moving, there is no place [in the body] that does not move. When still, there is no place that isn't still. First seek extension, then contraction; then it can be fine and subtle.[11]

> —Wu Yu-hsiang

---

9. This figure was reproduced from Edward R. Shaw, *Physics by Experiment*, 28.
10. https://en.wikipedia.org/wiki/Sarcomere.
11. Lo et al., *The Essence of T'ai Chi Ch'uan*, 57.

The above statement by Wu Yu-hsiang might be written as follows:

Remember, when a part of the body moves, every part of the body contributes to that movement by expanding and then condensing.

In the state of bodily unification achieved by expansion, a change in any part of the body will automatically affect every other part of the body. The concepts listed below express that idea. Interestingly, the first one is from physics (Pascal's principle again), and the others are from the Taijiquan Classics.

Any change in the pressure at any point in a confined liquid will result in the same change at all points in the liquid.

—Pascal's Principle

Remember, when moving, there is no place that doesn't move.[12]

—Wu Yu-hsiang

All parts of the body are strung together without the slightest break.[13]

—Chang San-feng

The whole body is a hand, and a hand is not a hand.[14]

—Cheng Man-ch'ing

The [nei] jin of the (whole) body, through practice becomes one unit.[15]

—Li I-yu

Because of the heightened alertness achieved in a state of bodily unification, you will be able to instantaneously move in any direction and exert actual strength in all directions.

Educating Bioelectrical Pathways

Imagining moving against resistance in practicing Taiji involves the constantly changing, moment-by-moment sending, receiving, and processing of electrical information. Doing so leads to educating bioelectrical pathways for coordinated, quick, efficient, and appropriate responses to new situations. Practicing

---

12. Lo et al., *The Essence of T'ai Chi Ch'uan*. 57.
13. Lo et al., *The Essence of T'ai Chi Ch'uan*, 24.
14. Lo et al., *The Essence of T'ai Chi Ch'uan*, 95.
15. Lo et al., *The Essence of T'ai Chi Ch'uan*, 76.

electrifying and expanding your limbs and trunk will increase your alertness and noticeably shorten your processing and response times.

A recent Harvard Medical School web article quotes a study showing that "Taiji can improve cognitive function."[16] Perhaps that study might show stronger results by grouping subjects by use of *nei jin* or not.

Consider the following passage from the Taiji Classics:

A feather cannot be added; nor can a fly alight.[17]

—Wang Tsung-yueh

This statement by Wang Tsung-yueh is usually taken to mean that the body should be so delicately balanced and free-moving that the addition of a feather will be felt for its weight and that a fly alighting will set the whole body into motion. Perhaps the meaning of Wang Tsung-yueh's statement can alternatively be taken to refer to what Professor Cheng says is the benefit of swimming on land: "Functionally, this slow movement against an imagined resistance will ultimately create great speed in responding to a fighting situation." That is, with continued practice, the bioelectrical pathways of expansive movement become so dependably established and ready to be activated that the slightest external stimulus is quickly processed, and the appropriate bodily response is instantaneous.

Deception in Self-Defense

In a self-defense situation, an opponent can easily read your intention if you use conventional (contractive) strength. Moreover, feeling your strength, the opponent then automatically increases his strength, and each party keeps escalating until the stronger one wins. But what if you are weakened by old age, injury, or illness? Then the opponent will probably be stronger than you and will likely win. On the other hand, the use of expansive strength is concealed and does not lead to such an escalation. If your *jin* [*nei jin*] is highly developed, an opponent who contacts you feels that your limbs are very heavy and connected to every other part of your body. Such strength is concealed and not easily read by the opponent, who doesn't tend to escalate his strength. Of course, expansive strength isn't enough—you also need to be trained in self-defense.

The opponent doesn't know me; I alone know him. To become a peerless boxer results from this.[18]

—Wang Tsung-yueh

---

16. https://www.health.harvard.edu/mind-and mood/a-sharper-mind-tai-chi-can-improve-cognitive-function.

17. Lee Ying-arng, *Lee's Modified Tai Chi for Health* (Honolulu, HI: Mclisa Enterprises, 1968), 39.

18. Lo et al., *The Essence of T'ai Chi Ch'uan*, 35.

Chapter 6
Health Protocols Using Expansion

Expansion for Reeducating Upper-Back Alignment

Kyphosis

Kyphosis (hunchbacked) is the medical term for an excessive rearward convexity of the thoracic spine. Having taught Taiji to seniors—some in their upper nineties—for the past two decades, I can say that there are few beyond seventy years of age who are exempt from kyphosis. Actually, many much-younger people suffer from varying degrees of this condition without even realizing it.

Causative factors are inadequate nutrients, improper bodily usage, and insufficient exercise, hydration, sleep, and exposure to sunlight.

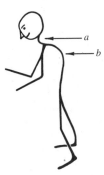

Fig. 6-1. A depiction of an excessive curvature of the upper back: (a) the cervical spine is excessively curved to reduce the downward aspect of the head, and (b) the excessive curve of the upper back. Hunching forward to this degree requires the use of a walker to support the body.

Those with severe kyphosis compensate for having their heads dipped forward by lifting their chins, thereby accentuating the curves in their necks

(Fig. 6-1). If this compensation is insufficient, the next way of compensating is to thrust their pelvises forward (Fig. 6-2).

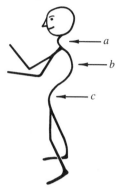

Fig. 6-2. A depiction of the results of compensating for an excessive curvature of the upper back: (*a*) the cervical spine is excessively curved to reduce the downward aspect of the head, and (*c*) the pelvis is thrust forward, allowing the body to be more balanced and upright at the expense of an excessively curved lower back.

My Struggle with Kyphosis

I started to develop a serious kyphosis when in my teens, possibly from practicing the piano while hunched forward for hours on a daily basis. When I was in my twenties, my kyphosis had progressed to the point where I experienced severe pain that was relieved only by lying on my back for a while.

One day in the 1970s, when I was lying on my back on the floor of an empty classroom to relieve my pain, one of my high school students, Kate Antrobus, noticed and asked me what was wrong. When I told her, she said, "You should go to my teacher, Elaine Summers. She is a genius. She can help you." Whereas massage, chiropractic, meditation, and Taiji reduced the pain, their benefit to my excessive back curvature was minimal. So I was somewhat skeptical but decided to keep an open mind and contact Summers.

The progress I made under Summers's system, Kinetic Awareness® (KA), was substantial. My excessive spinal curvature and the resulting pain were lessened, and the changes I made during each weekly session with her were evident.

In recent years, I have been delving deeper into the problem of forward spinal curvature and have found that applying Summers's concept of frontal expansion has had impressive effects, not only for myself but for a number of the students in their eighties and nineties to whom I teach Taiji.

Causes of Kyphosis

Consider young people whose spinal alignment hasn't been corrupted by doing repeated, lengthy tasks wherein their bodies are leaning forward. For them, all vertebrae are balanced without any need for muscular tension to maintain the natural spinal curves in a relaxed alignment.

However, we tend to bend forward much more often than backward. We sit at desks, use computers and "smart" phones, read, play keyboard instruments, and sit on furniture at home and in transportation that encourages us to slouch. After long periods of our habitually leaning forward, the disks, which separate adjacent vertebrae, become misshapen. The vertebrae also may lose bone in the front. The result is a forward curvature of the spine. Next, strength must be used to maintain correct alignment. But contractive strength of the back muscles can only be maintained for a short time. At a certain point, effort to try to maintain correct alignment becomes futile because the back muscles are in a state of trauma. "Standing up straight" is then painful, and the back muscles surrender and become flaccid. Over time, those muscles lengthen under the strain, and the condition escalates to a degree based on their strength and tone.

Adverse Effects of Kyphosis

There are adverse effects beyond the pain of the muscles in the upper back, which are stretched to their limit. One such effect is that the lungs, heart, and digestive organs are compressed. Another effect is that eventually spinal openings through which nerves emerge from the spine are reduced, thereby pinching and inflaming nerves, resulting in secondary pain.

Advice Often Given for Reversing Kyphosis

The frequent advice for those with an excessive forward spinal curvature is, "Stand up straight, pull your shoulders back, and pull your chin in." Whereas these actions may be somewhat beneficial in strengthening and toning the muscles involved, it is not a realistic solution to the problem because it is impossible for muscular contraction of the back muscles to hold the spine in an optimal posture for more than a short time—if at all. Thus, using the back muscles to support spinal alignment is not useful in reversing the problem and does not get to its root cause.

Expansion of the front of the trunk of the body can make a big difference in supporting spinal alignment. Practicing upward and lateral expansion of the front of the chest can slow down or even arrest the progression of the forward curvature. In some cases, the excessive curvature can be somewhat reversed.

A Protocol for Arresting or Reversing Kyphosis

The following protocol can provide three possible levels of success: (1) the kyphosis decreases, (2) it does not decrease or worsen, and (3) it worsens but at a slower rate than otherwise. Levels (1) and (2) can reduce pain and some of the harmful effects. In my experience, it is possible to achieve level (1).

The protocol has two parts: (1) learning to expand and open the front of the trunk of the body to provide support and prevent it from collapsing and (2) strengthening and toning the back muscles—not so that they can support alignment but so they can begin to attain a more-normal length and tone.

Supporting the Front Through Expansion. The goal is to recognize and produce expansion of the front of the body in every direction. With practice over time, it becomes natural to maintain that state without conscious thought or effort. Two typical exercises are shown below.

One valuable exercise is to stand facing the corner of a room, place one hand on each adjacent wall a comfortable distance apart (Fig. 6-3). Then slowly move the body forward, expanding the front and relaxing the back at the same time. Here gravity is playing a small but useful part. It is essential that any forward movement be accompanied by an active opening of the front of the body.

Another exercise is to stand, tilting slightly forward, with the outer edges of your hands resting on a large ball. Then slowly roll the ball up the wall, at the same time actively expanding the front and relaxing the back (Fig. 6-4).

Other Exercises Involving Expansion. Most movements of the Taiji empty-hand form involve alternately opening and closing parts of the body. In some movements, the opening and closing is subtle and might easily go unnoticed. In other movements such as "Single Whip," "White Crane," and "Diagonal Flying," the opening and closing is dramatic. It is of great value to recognize the extent to which the condensing and expanding the front of the body contributes to the arm movements. Of course, each movement has a slightly different direction of the opening and closing. For example, "Cloud Hands," as done in the Cheng Man-ch'ing style, has a vertical opening and closing of the front of the body. "White Crane," "Diagonal Flying," and "Deflect Downward, Parry, and Punch" provide diagonal openings and closings. Other movements have various combinations of opening and closing in different ways.

Most of the Taiji movements involve stepping, which makes it harder to discern the extent to which you may be condensing and expanding. However, there is one section of the form, "Grasping the Sparrow's Tail," that involves a succession of movements requiring no stepping, namely, "Ward off Right," "Roll Back and Press," and "Withdraw and Push." These movements are ideal for isolating the practice of expanding and condensing.

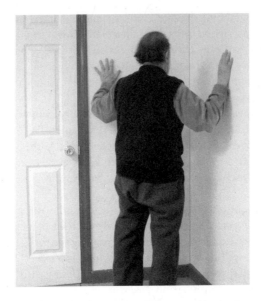

Fig. 6-3. The author facing a 90-degree corner of the room, with a hand on each adjacent wall, actively expanding the front of his body to open it.

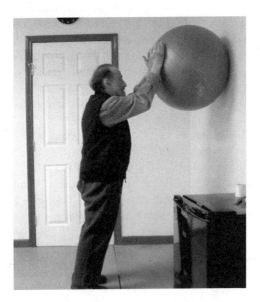

Fig. 6-4. The author rolling a large ball up the wall to open the front of his body as it actively expands.

I also find that elements of the "Turtle Qigong"[1] provide an excellent opportunity to practice expanding and condensing the front of the body in different ways.

Strength Training. Training the contractive strength of the back muscles is very important, not because doing so itself reverses kyphosis. The reason for such strengthening is that, as support of the front of the body arising from expansion allows the back muscles to relax, they will be more apt to regain their tone and more correct length. Moreover, the stronger the back muscles are, the less susceptible they will be to excessive lengthening when frontal support is lacking.

The back-strengthening exercises shown in Figures 6-5 and 6-6 should also be done with active expansion of the front of the body when pulling back (Fig. 6-5) and when opening (Fig. 6-6). Condensing of the front should occur during the release part of the movement.

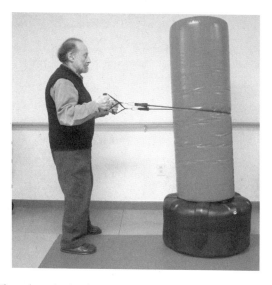

Fig. 6-5. The author using bands to strengthen his back muscles by pulling back. Active expansion is used for opening the front of the body, and contraction is used for the back.

---

1. https://www.youtube.com/watch?v=ZOhoUyxIgaU.

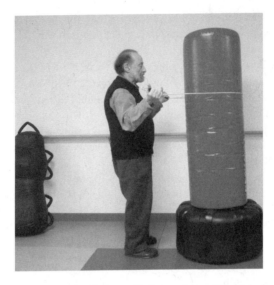

Fig. 6-6. The author using bands to open his front and strengthen his back muscles by separating his chest and arms laterally. Expansion is used for the front of the body, and contraction is used for the back.

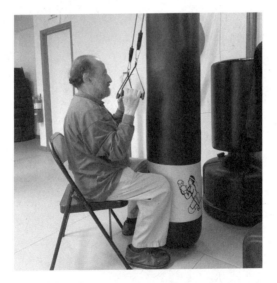

Fig. 6-7. The author using bands to strengthen his back muscles by pulling downward, elbows inward. The bands are draped around the chains supporting the bag from the ceiling.

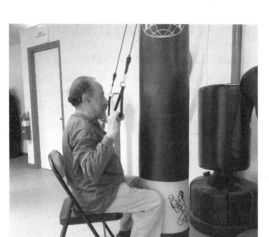

Fig. 6-8. The author using bands to strengthen his back muscles by pulling downward, elbows outward.

Two additional strengthening exercises are shown in Figures 6-7 and 6-8. As you pull downward, you also extend the spine upward.

Utilizing Movements of the Taiji Form for Arresting or Reversing Kyphosis

Each movement of the form is suitable for practicing expansion of the front of the body, but some movements, such as "Beginning," "Withdraw and Push," "Single Whip," and "White Crane" are particularly suitable.

> **Experiment 6-1.** After the initial lifting of your arms and extending the palms of the hands in "Beginning," lower your arms, keeping your forearms level. In lowering, let gravity move your arms back and downward by releasing your shoulders so that your elbows arc downward and backward rather than pulling them backward. Recognize that doing so opens the front of your body. Then actively augment that opening using expansive strength.

> **Experiment 6-2.** As the arms separate and move rearward in "Withdraw and Push," again recognize that doing so opens the front of the body. Then actively augment that opening using expansive strength.

Expansion for Reeducating the Lower Back

Causes of Excessive Lower-Back Curvature

Many people—especially women—experience lower-back problems. Such problems can result from lifting heavy objects improperly, being overweight, and copying adults with poor posture, starting when very young. Another detrimental, excessive inward curvature of the lower back lorfdosis often originates from heels on shoes, which unnaturally lift the backs of the legs, causing the body to tilt forward. To compensate for the tilt, the top of the body must lean backward, thus harmfully accentuating the lumbar curve of the spine ("swayback") (see Fig. 6-9).

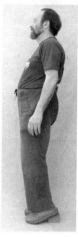

Fig. 6-9. A simulation of the harmful postural effects of heels on shoes. Note how the pelvis is thrust forward, causing the inward curve of the lower back to be unnaturally exaggerated.[2]

An excessive lumbar curve undermines the alignment of the entire spine and causes other problems, including lower-back pain. My book *Tai Chi Dynamics* has a section on *han xiong ba bei* (hollow the chest and expand the back) and how expansive strength plays a role.[3] I explain by means of force diagrams how an excessive lumbar curve makes the body weak, how using contraction makes the body weak, but how using expansive strength makes the body strong.

Unfortunately, *han xiong ba bei* is sometimes misinterpreted by Taiji practitioners and teachers to mean "tuck the tailbone forward," which indirectly forces the lumbar curve to be reduced. However, reducing that curve

2. This photo was reproduced from Robert Chuckrow, *Tai Chi Walking* (Wolfeboro, NH: YMAA Publication Center, 2002), 21.

3. Robert Chuckrow, *Tai Chi Dynamics* (Wolfeboro, NH: YMAA Publication Center, 2008), 93–94, 96–97.

by tucking, which pits one part of the body against another, goes against the Taiji principles and is a harmful, unnatural way of treating the body. There is a big difference between (a) achieving *han xiong ba bei* by sending bioelectrical messages to extend the muscles that control the lumbar curve and (b) forcing the lumbar spine into place by means of contracting muscles that are in a different part of the body.

Experiment 6-3. Learning to Expand Your Lower Back. You will need a pillow and a small towel. The height of the pillow should be such that when you lie on your back with your head on the pillow, your cervical spine is in its optimal alignment. Roll up the towel. Lie on the floor with the towel under your lower back and your head on the pillow. Start by surrendering to gravity, relaxing every part of your body. Relaxation is essential to achieving an awareness of what parts are involved in activating a movement. Next, gently press your lower back into the towel by using the muscles around the part of the spine touching the towel. Only a tiny amount of movement is necessary. There may be a tendency to use other parts such as your abdomen, ribs, pelvis, or legs. However, the goal is to use only the muscles that are involved, namely those around that part of the spine.

If you habitually accentuate the curve in your lower back, this problem may involve your lack of awareness that you are overusing the associated muscles. If so, the object is to gain this awareness. After a while, try lifting your lower back away from the towel slightly. Then try arching your spine to one side and then the other slightly.

When you feel that you want to stop, rest until the changes in your body subside. Then roll over onto one side, and using your arms, come up sideways to a sitting position. This way of rising off the floor minimizes tensing the muscles around the spine and reverting to your habitual way of using those muscles. Then slowly come up to standing and feel your whole body. It is also useful to recreate that heavy feeling you get after taking a hot bath.

It may take some time to learn how to move your lumbar spine independently, but once you have learned to do so, you will become aware of habitual tension in that region and have the tools to release it.

Tucking the Tailbone in Taiji-Form Practice: Good or Bad?

Of course, *releasing* the tailbone is good. But some Yoga and Taiji teachers erroneously tell students to *tuck* their tailbones to reduce an excessive curvature of the lumbar spine. Doing so fails to get to the root of the problem and adds an additional problem of one set of muscles bullying another.

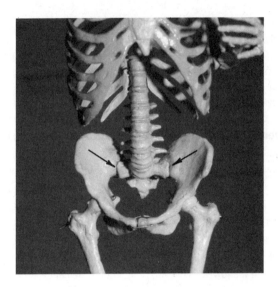

Fig. 6-10. Front view of the sacroiliac joints (located at arrow heads), joining each side of the sacrum with the pelvis.

One problem is that many who try to tuck their tailbones do so by tilting their pelvis forward, which alone does not really help straighten the lumbar spine. A look at an anatomical drawing of the pelvis and spine will reveal that they are interconnected by the sacroiliac joints. Those joints provide an independent rotational movement; namely, the pelvis can tilt forward and backward without the spine having any movement (Fig. 6-10).

Whereas titling the pelvis can have value as an exercise, holding the pelvis in a fixed alignment for an extended period cuts off blood and *qi*.

Experiment 6-4. Checking Independence of Motion of Pelvis and Spine. While standing, place the forefinger of one hand on your tailbone (sacrum), and tilt your pelvis forward and backward. Notice that the movement of the pelvis need not cause any movement of the sacrum.

Tilting the tailbone to force the lumbar spine to straighten requires holding bones in place by means of sustained contraction of one group of muscles against that of an opposing group. Pitting two muscle groups against each another exacerbates and does not get to the root of the problem, which is using sustained contractive muscular force to produce the excessive curve. The appropriate way of releasing this frozen tension is to become aware of it and do small, mindful, relaxed movements that enable awareness of habitually pulling your spine out of its optimal alignment (Experiment 6-2).

Important: Extending the tailbone downward is beneficial as is extending any part of the body. Extending the tailbone is entirely different from tucking it. Just as the head is said to be extended upward, which really means extending the cervical spine to the atlas, which supports the head, the lumbar spine also must be extended downward. Doing so is often a missing link in expansion and produces a substantial increase in rooting and the exertion of expansive strength. It should be noted that bones are incapable of moving on their own but be moved by the contraction of muscles or the expansion of surrounding tissues

How the Taiji Principles and Philosophy Apply

The most basic Taiji principle is that of the separation of *yin* and *yang*. The front of the body is *yin*, the back is *yang*. The *yang* elements that apply are active, expanded, and convex. The *yin* elements that apply are inactive, supportive, and concave. Tucking the tailbone requires contracting the front, which reverses *yin* and *yang*; that is, the front becomes active (*yang*), and the back becomes inactive (*yin*). Moreover, the Taiji principles teach us not to force anything and to have every joint in its most neutral alignment. For example, the Taiji Classics say, "In any action, the whole body must be made as light and free-moving as possible, so light that the addition of a feather will be felt for its weight, and so free-moving that a fly cannot alight on it without setting it in motion." Fixating the tailbone, pelvis, and hip joints in an off-centered alignment is antithetical to the basic principles of Taiji.

A preferred way to work on a person's excessive lumbar curvature is through experiments that reveal to the person that he or she is using a lot of muscular tension to sustain the excessive curvature. Once that habitual muscular tension is released, the spine at least has a chance of gradually assuming its natural shape.

I have successfully worked with a number of students on this issue over the years. The critical stage is to learn to expand the muscles of the lower back. My experience is that most people require quite a bit of instruction and practice in this regard.

Whereas it is important to be able to attain a state of *han xiong ba bei* when it is needed for exerting a large forward force, doing the form in a such a continued state of extension has no purpose because you are not exerting a large force on another person. The natural lumbar curve is appropriate for standing and locomoting, as occurs in the movements of the Taiji form. Holding the body in a state of unnecessary tension is a fixation, which is also against the Taiji principles. Instead, in doing the Taiji form, it is only necessary to allow the pelvis to float and the lumbar curve and tailbone to release naturally. Of course, those practitioners who are unable to achieve *han xiong ba bei* without tucking their tailbones will need to retrain their thinking and learn to attain a natural, released shape of their lumbar spines.

Improving the Cervical Spine Using Slow, Relaxed Movement

One of the Kinetic Awareness® activities that Elaine Summers taught me is extremely effective for relieving tension in the neck. It is also very simple and meditative. KA emphasizes relying on oneself as much as possible and getting to the root of a problem by doing simple movements very slowly and mindfully. Doing so enables you to discover pockets of tension which can be relieved by (a) your expectation that that tension will dissolve and (b) passive, relaxed, slow, meditative movement. KA movement is often done while lying on the floor, where not having to deal with gravity and balance enables you to relax as much as possible and to release your preconceptions about how your body should move.

Experiment 6-5. Relaxing Neck Muscles. For the following experiment, you will need an area of wood or carpeted floor large enough to lie on and an air-filled rubber or plastic ball about three to four inches in diameter. So much the better if the ball is somewhat dead. You can also use a pillow instead of a ball.

Lie down on your back (you can lie on an exercise mat if you want), and place the ball under the back of your head in such a manner that the center of your head is directly over the center of the ball and your head is centered (turned neither to the right or left) relative to your body (see Fig. 6-11).

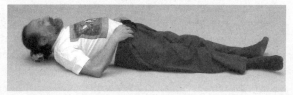

Fig. 6-11. Centered position of head on ball

Lie still for a while with your head resting on the ball, surrendering to gravity and releasing as much tension as possible everywhere in your body. It may take quite some time to begin to discover tension, some of which is so habitual that it can persist unrecognized for long periods of time—hours, days, weeks, months, and even years. Such tension is difficult to release without

(continued on next page)

---

movement. Doing movement so slowly that you can become aware of the muscular action involved enables you to release muscles that are in a state of self-perpetuating excess tension. At the same time, blood can transport oxygen and nutrients into the affected cells and flush toxic waste products out. The slow, relaxed movement also increases the flow of *qi*.

Once you have achieved a sufficient state of relaxation, start turning your head to the side extremely slowly and continuously, relaxing every muscle in your body as much as possible as you move. The movement should be done so slowly and continuously that only an adept observer will be able to detect any motion.

Important: If you experience any pain during the movement, do not proceed. Instead, take time to work on relaxing the muscles involved so that you can ease through painlessly. Doing an otherwise painful movement painlessly produces the most-therapeutic result.

As you turn your head, there will be a tendency for it to roll off the ball. Therefore, either keep the center of your head directly over that of the ball as you turn, or reposition the ball using your hands, which is okay as long as repositioning is not done so frequently that it prevents experiencing a quasi-meditative state.

When your head reaches the end of its natural motion (Fig. 6-12), dwell in that position, continuing to release as much tension as possible. When you have succeeded in surrendering to gravity sufficiently, move back to center in the same relaxed, slow, and continuous manner, and rest and feel the effect. When changes in your body subside, repeat on the other side.

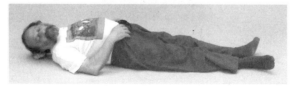

Fig. 6-12. Turned position of head on ball.

When you are finished, you can rest with your head resting on the ball in its centered orientation.

Caution: If you feel yourself drifting asleep or entering a meditative state, remove the ball to prevent your head rolling off it and hitting the floor. To optimize the alignment of your cervical spine, you can do this exercise with your head resting on the floor or on a pillow of an appropriate height instead

(continued on next page)

of on a ball. Also, keep in mind that it is cooler on the floor than higher up, so you may want a blanket to cover your body.

When you are done, roll onto your side. Then with continuous movement, slowly come to sitting or standing, using your arms to lift you rather than unnecessarily tensing the muscles around the spine, which you have just worked on relaxing.

Alternatively, you can do Experiment 6-5 with the ball under the back of your neck instead of under the back of your head.

Expansion for Relieving Plantar Fasciitis

Plantar fasciitis is an inflammation of a thick band of tissue that connects the heel bone to the toes on the sole of the foot. It is a condition wherein pain is experienced on one or both soles between the arch and the heel.

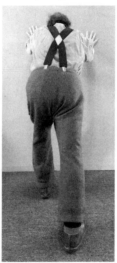

Fig. 6-13. A counterproductive way of stretching by using gravity and leverage to lengthen the muscles of the back of the leg. The sole of the foot is also being stretched, which can increase its inflammation.

In my experience, a cause of plantar fasciitis is over-stretching the sole of the foot by pushing downward with the ball of the foot and raising the heel repetitively or continually for too long a time. My original bout of plantar fasciitis occurred just after doing Baguazhang circle-walking totally on the balls of my feet. The pain on both of my feet lasted for six months. It flared up again after standing for too long on the balls of my feet on the narrow rungs of a ladder.

One conventional protocol involves sitting and pulling the foot toward you with a towel whose middle is looped around the ball of the foot and whose ends are held in both hands. Another counterproductive stretching exercise is shown in Figure 6-13. From my experience, it is inappropriate to use leverage, gravity, or an opposing set of muscles to stretch inflamed tissues.

Instead of stretching the tissues on the sole of the foot, it is preferable to stand with the ball of the affected foot on the tread of a flight of stairs, with the heel hanging beyond the tread. Then extend the heel downward by extending the muscles on the back of the lower leg rather than by mercilessly stretching the tissues on the sole of the foot (Fig. 6-14). Extending the hamstrings and calf muscles relieves the pull of those muscles on the heel of the foot and, consequently, on the sole. In the incipient stages of the return of plantar fasciitis, this protocol provides immediate relief.

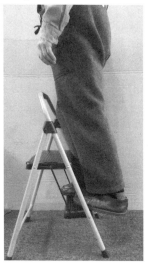

Fig. 6-14. A recommended way of stretching to relieve plantar fasciitis. In this case, the heel is extended downward with the sole of the foot relaxed.

Chapter 7
Balance

Balance depends on many elements, some of which are herein discussed: 1) gravity; 2) leg strength; 3) an awareness of the pressure distribution on the soles of the feet; 4) knee, ankle, arch alignment; 5) center of mass; 6) range of motion throughout the body; 7) vision; 8) awareness of your surroundings and limitations; and 9) a brief mention of the semicircular canals.

Gravity

The Riddle of the Sphinx

In the Ancient Greek play, *Oedipus Rex*, by Sophocles (c. 496–c. 406 BCE), Oedipus succeeded in solving the riddle of the Sphinx: "What walks on four legs in the morning, two legs at noon, and three legs in the evening?" The answer is "Man." Humans start off crawling on all fours, then walk upright, but finally succumb to gravity later in life and must walk with a cane.

The force of gravity is our friend—without it we would float helplessly. But we must constantly contend with it. Many seniors are concerned about falling, and fatality after a fall increases with age. Practicing Taiji improves balance and reduces the chance of falling and also of being injured from falling. Of course, the probability of falling can be further reduced when a comprehension of the mechanics of balance is brought into Taiji movement and daily life.

Rooting and Balance

Rooting means being connected to the ground like a tree whose roots are deeply embedded in the earth. Two main goals in martial-arts practice are to be rooted and to be skilled in "breaking the root" of an opponent. Losing a connection to the ground can have serious consequences in martial arts as well as daily life.

Rooting and *Song*

Song (Chapter 1) is one of the most important conditions for rooting. As soon as tension develops—especially in your upper body—not only is your root undermined, but your center of mass rises, thereby increasing the chance of injury from a fall (center of mass is discussed later in this chapter).

Song is also necessary for achieving expansive strength (Chapter 2), which is important for effective power and bodily resilience. Finally, *song* results in the center of gravity being much lower, which means increased stability and less injury should a fall occur.

Leg Strength and Mobility

When you begin to lose your balance—even to a small degree—shifting your weight is often a factor in recovering stability. So a combination of mobility and leg strength is important in preventing falling. The stronger your legs and the greater their range of motion, the greater the ability to correct for a loss of balance.

There have been a number of studies reporting that seniors and those with health issues such as Parkinson's disease fall less frequently as a result of studying Taiji. This conclusion agrees with the experience of some of my students who are seniors. The question is, what is it about Taiji that reduces falls?

Many seniors—and even younger people—are susceptible to falls because they spend a lot of time sitting, which causes their leg muscles to atrophy. The increase in leg strength produced by practicing Taiji helps substantially. Taiji stepping involves having the weight on a stationary leg while it is bent much more than is required in daily life. The resulting stretch of the quadriceps and other muscles in the legs not only increases adaptive ability but also results in a substantial increase in leg strength.

Exercises for Strengthening Leg Muscles

Here are a few valuable exercises for strengthening calves and quadriceps.

Heel-Circling. This exercise was taught by Professor Cheng for helping a knee injury heal. It is also very valuable for strengthening the quadriceps muscle. This is not a balance exercise, so lightly hold onto something stable. Then start by standing on one leg (Fig. 7-1). Bend the rooted leg and lift the knee of the empty leg. Then, without lowering the knee, extend the heel outward and then down in an arc. Repeat a few times, then kick your leg to release the muscles. After resting, do the other side. Over time, as your leg strength allows, increase the number of repetitions on each side to a total of thirty-six times in a row.

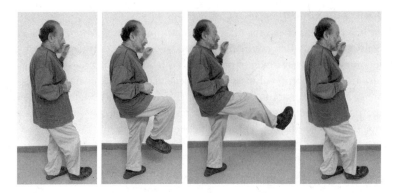

Fig. 7-1. The heel-circling exercise shown by Cheng Man-ch'ing.

Leg-Lifting. Sit in a chair, lift one leg, and extend it horizontally, tightening the quadriceps. Then rest and repeat. Start with only a few repetitions and increase only as your leg strength increases. Make sure you always do both sides.

Body Lifts. Hold onto something stable. Then lift one leg. Rise onto the ball of the rooted foot and lower the heel. Start with only a few repetitions and increase the number of repetitions only as your leg strength increases. Make sure you always do both sides. Eventually, you can increase the intensity of this exercise with the ball of your foot on a stair tread, each time lowering your heel below the level of the tread.

Caution: Overdoing this exercise can lead to plantar fasciitis, an inflammation of the fascia of sole of the foot. So take it slowly.

Increasing Mobility

Over the decades that I have been teaching Taiji, I start every class with a warm-up and some meditative stretching. I have observed over this time that few people of all ages can even get close to touching their toes. Most utilize upper-back mobility rather than that of their hamstrings.

There are many ways of stretching. The way I have found that provides the best combination of progress, safety, and healthful byproducts is by using expansion and gravity rather than pitting one part of the body against another.[1]

---

1. For a video of the author's general stretching routine, visit https://www.chuckrowtaichi.com/StretchingRoutine.html.

Experiment 7-1. A useful stretching exercise involves letting the body hang from the hip joints with legs slightly bent (Fig. 7-2). It is important to extend the hip joints upward, relax, and feel the weight of every part of the body above the hip joints, and shift the weight forward onto the balls of the feet without clenching the toes. A common practice is lifting and then lowering the body, with the goal of lowering further each time. There are two ways to lift the hanging body.

The active way of lifting involves contracting the hamstrings and back muscles. This way is counterproductive because it tightens and shortens the muscles we are endeavoring to relax and lengthen. The passive (and better) way of lifting is to inhale, causing the lower abdomen to expand against the fronts of the thighs, thereby lifting the body without contracting the back muscles and hamstrings. The exhalation then further releases those muscles and lowers you more than the inhalation raised you.

Repeat this way of raising and lowering three times.

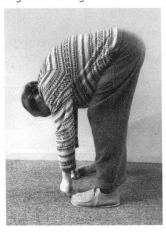

Fig. 7-2. The body hanging from the hip joints with legs slightly bent.

Note: It is important to rise from hanging without contracting your hamstrings or back muscles for the following reasons: (1) Tensing the very muscles you have just worked on relaxing deprives you of experiencing them in their relaxed state when you come up. (2) Muscles can become traumatized when coaxed into an unaccustomed length and then suddenly forced to contract under load. They need time to recover their tone. (3) Rising by using your back muscles puts a large, potentially injurious stress on your spine as would lifting a heavy, external object that way.

(continued on next page)

Instead, come up by simultaneously bending your knees, dropping your tail-bone, and bringing the trunk of your body to almost vertical while flexing your spine as little as possible. Then rise vertically by straightening your legs. You should lift your body in the same way as you would lift a heavy object—with your legs, not your back.

An additional non-passive but valuable action to do while hanging is to lift one hip joint and lower the other one. Then alternately change each side's role. The lifting action occurs by extending the muscles on the back of a leg rather than contracting the muscles in front. That way, the hamstrings and back muscles lengthen on their own terms instead of by being forced to do so by the opposing muscles.

Finding the Centers of the Feet

The following experiments, spawned by training I received from Sam Chin Fan-siong, are extremely valuable.

Rocking Forward and Backward

Experiment 7-2. Stand in a 50-50 stance (weight 50 percent on each foot), with feet parallel and a comfortable distance apart. *Feet parallel* means that the centerlines of the feet should be parallel.

Shift the weight forward onto the balls of your feet, then rock backward until you are on your heels. Keep rocking forward and backward, realizing that during each cycle, the pressure alternates between forward of and behind the lateral (left/right) centerline of each foot (Fig. 7-3). Then reduce the amplitude of each excursion, each time passing the center until you end up on the lateral centerlines of your feet. That is, the distribution of pressure on each foot is then centered on its lateral centerline. Capture that feeling so you can recreate it later.

Alternately Rocking to the Outsides and Insides of Your Feet

Stand in a 50-50 stance. Bring your knees outward, thereby shifting the weight onto the outsides of your feet. Then bring your knees inward, thereby shifting the weight onto the insides of your feet. Keep shifting from one side to the other, realizing that during each cycle, the pressure on each foot moves side to side, crossing its median centerline of each foot. Then reduce the amplitude of each excursion, each time crossing the median (forward) centerlines of your feet until you end up on their median centerlines. Capture that feeling so you can recreate it later.

Now repeat both directions, forward/backward and sideways, until you can stand with the pressure distribution on each foot centered on the intersection of the two centerlines you just located.

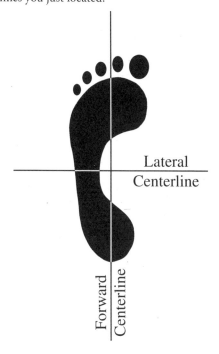

Fig. 7-3. The forward and lateral centerlines of the foot. The center of the foot is the intersection of these centerlines. Note that for the foot shown, there is zero pressure on the center of the foot.

Locating the Centers of the Feet

The center of the foot is the intersection of the forward and lateral centerlines (see Fig. 7-3). In this figure, the forward centerline passes between the second and third toes. This relationship, which requires the use of vision and the analytical mind, is only a rough guide and not meant to substitute for the direct experience provided by the rocking exercises in Experiment 7-2.

Consider the following points:

• Making any change to a habitual pattern will feel strange.

• During Taiji practice—or daily life, for that matter—recreate the feeling of the pressure distribution on each foot centered on that foot for each step.

- The center of your foot might have little or no pressure even though the distribution of your full weight is centered there.

- Whatever the amount of weight on a foot, the pressure distribution on that foot should be centered on that foot.

During stepping, the weight is 100 percent on one foot. A foot is only several inches wide, so a small lateral inaccuracy of the distribution of weight on it can cause a loss of balance. When the weight distribution shifts to the outside of the foot, little strength exists for restoring balance. When it shifts to the inside of a foot, the help of the big toe in regaining balance may be unreliable.

In a two-person situation, when the weight distribution goes to your heels, you are susceptible to being pushed, and when it goes to the balls of your feet, you are susceptible to being pulled forward.

Knee, Ankle, Arch Alignment

Correct knee, ankle, and arch alignment has become increasingly emphasized by Taiji teachers. When the alignment of the legs, ankles, and feet is off, there is a tendency to avoid putting weight on the legs; after all, poor alignment is potentially injurious, and the body resists sinking into a leg that is malaligned. Thus, the strength and mobility of the legs is undermined by wrong alignment.[2]

Note: Having the weight on each foot centered is also helpful in attaining proper knee, ankle, and arch alignment. Such alignment is the topic of a whole chapter in *Tai Chi Walking*.[3]

If alignment is off, the need to suddenly shift onto one foot to avoid falling can result in a painful injury to the knee or ankle and then cause a worse fall.

Shifting Your Weight from One Foot to the Other

Experiment 7-3. Stand in a 50-50 stance, with feet shoulder width apart. The centerlines of the feet should be parallel.

Next, slowly shift your weight onto one foot, keeping the pressure distribution on each foot centered as you do so. Because you are continually sustaining a centered pressure distribution on each foot, when the weight shifts to 100 percent on one foot, the pressure distribution on that foot will automatically be on center, with no adjustment needed.

Then slowly shift back to the other foot, and alternately shift side-to-side, making sure that as you do so, the pressure distribution on each foot remains centered.

---

2. Also see https://chuckrowtaichi.com/Alignment.html for a treatment of knee, ankle, and arch alignment.

3. Robert Chuckrow, *Tai Chi Walking* (Wolfeboro, NH: YMAA Publication Center, 2002), Ch. 3.

Experiment 7-4. Stand in a 70-30 stance such that the pressure distribution on each foot is centered (Fig. 7-4).

Next, slowly shift your weight onto your rear foot in such a way that the pressure on each foot is continually centered. When the weight becomes 100 percent on one foot, the pressure distribution on that foot will automatically be on center.

Then slowly shift back to having 70 percent of the weight on the forward foot, and alternately shift forward and backward.

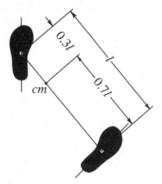

Fig. 7-4. A 70-30 stance. Note that the center of mass (*cm*) of the body is directly over the straight line joining the centers of the feet, 70 percent of the way from the center of the rear foot to that of the front foot.[4]

Circling Your Knees

Experiment 7-5. Stand with your feet parallel, a comfortable distance apart (Fig. 7-5). Bend your knees about halfway and circle them, keeping the center of the pressure distribution on each foot centered.

Note: The goal is to have the pressure distribution on each foot always centered. It is, however, very difficult if not impossible to be conscious of more than one thing at the same time. So, at first, shift your awareness from one foot to the other and make corrections. With continued practice, your subconscious mind will take over and do the job effortlessly.

---

4. Note that the line joining the centers of the feet is not necessarily perpendicular to the centerline of the rear foot although it is close to perpendicular in this diagram. Variables are the shoulder width of the person involved, how far the forward foot has stepped, and how much the rear foot is turned in.

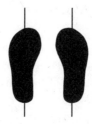

Fig. 7-5. A fairly close 50-50 stance, with the centerlines of the feet parallel. Note that the center of mass of your body is directly over the point midway between the centers of the feet.

Center of Mass

The center of mass (*cm*) of an object is a point at which the object is in balance when freely supported there. The center of mass of a symmetric, homogeneous object is at its geometric center. Also, based on an object's shape, its center of mass need not even be located on that object. For example, the center of mass of a flat washer is located at its geometric center, within its central hole (Fig. 7-6).

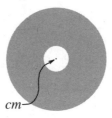

cm

Fig. 7-6. The center of mass of a flat washer is located at its geometric center, within its central hole.

When a body is supported at any point and allowed to hang from that point so it can rotate freely, its center of mass will end up directly below that point. Thus, the center of mass of a two-dimensional (plane) object can be found as follows: suspend the object by any point *A* on it. The center of mass will then settle on a vertical line *l* through *A*. Then suspend the object by a different point *B* on it. The center of mass will then be on a vertical line *l'* through *B*. The intersection of *l* and *l'* is the center of mass. To check, suspend the object by a third point *C* on it. A vertical line *l"* will also intersect the center of mass (Fig. 7-7).

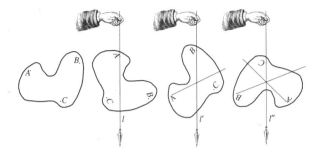

Fig. 7-7. The center of mass of a two-dimensional (plane) object is the intersection of two or more vertical lines *l*, *l'*, and *l"* through different freely supported points *A*, *B*, and *C*, respectively.

Center of Mass of a Person

The center of mass of a person is thought to be at the *dan tian*, a point one inch below the navel and one-third of the way from front to back. Because people can change their shape, their centers of mass can change with movement. For example, if you are standing on one leg in a balanced condition and move your other leg forward, that action brings your center of mass forward. If you do not adjust to that change, your balance will be off, and you will need to quickly lower that foot to the ground to avoid falling. Therefore, in order to maintain stability, it is necessary to compensate for this forward change by shifting your body correspondingly in the opposite direction to that of the extended leg so that your new center of mass will be directly above the center of the weighted foot. Experiments for this concept will be provided later in this chapter.

Visualizing Your Center of Mass

Now try redoing Experiments 7-3 and 7-4, this time visualizing your center of mass moving directly above the line joining the centers of your feet as you shift your weight.

> **Experiment 7-6.** Standing in a 50-50 stance, first visualize the line joining the centers of your feet (Fig. 7-8). Then recognize that the center of mass of your body is now on the midpoint of that line. Now shift your weight 100 percent onto one foot and then 100 percent to the other, visualizing your center of mass moving along that line, continually maintaining the pressure distribution on each foot centered on that foot.

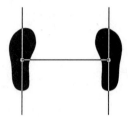

Fig. 7-8. A 50-50 shoulder-width stance, with the centerlines of the feet parallel. The horizontal line shown joins the centers of the feet.

Experiment 7-7. Stand in a 70-30 stance (Fig. 7-4). First visualize the line joining the centerlines of your feet. Note that the center of mass of your body is now on the line joining the centers of your feet, 70 percent of the way from the center of the rear foot to that of the front foot. Then slowly shift your weight 100 percent onto your rear foot and then back to 70 percent to the front foot. Visualize your center of mass moving directly above and along the line joining the centers of your feet, continually maintaining the pressure distribution on each foot centered on that foot.

As soon as your center of mass leaves the line joining the centers of your feet, the pressure distribution on one or both feet is then off center. As long as the pressure distribution on each foot is centered on that foot, the center of mass of your body is automatically directly over the line joining the centers of your feet.

Note: One of the benefits of practicing push-hands is developing the ability to extend your awareness beyond yourself and perceive the state of another. An experienced practitioner can instantly feel the center of mass of another and use it advantageously.

Balance Experiments

Balancing on One Leg

When you lift a leg to step in any direction, the weight and leverage of the lifted leg shifts your center of mass in the direction of that leg. In order to maintain balance on the other (rooted) leg, it is necessary to move the rest of your body a corresponding amount in the opposite direction in order to maintain your center of mass directly over the center of your weighted foot. Otherwise, your balance will be off.

Experiment 7-8. Place one foot at 45 degrees to the direction you are facing. Then slowly lift the other foot. As you do so, strive to maintain the pressure distribution centered on the rooted foot. Then move the free leg all the ways that you can—up, down, left, right behind, across, etc. As you move your free leg and turn your body, adjust your center of mass to be directly over the center of your rooted foot. It is important to realize that we tend to emphasize the active (*yang*) leg rather than the rooted (*yin*) one. So attend to the rooted foot and adjust the center of mass to be centered over the center of that foot as you move the active foot. When you tire, shake the rooted leg and change sides.

Note: It is important to do the following experiments very slowly so that you can be aware of every necessary change. Also, it is important to realize that we tend to overemphasize the moving (*yang*) leg, so it is good to be more aware of the rooted (*yin*) leg and its connection to the ground.

Experiment 7-9. Stand in the 50-50 stance of the outset of "Preparation" (Fig.7-9). Feel half of your weight centered on each foot. Shift and sink to the right, at the same time turning to the right. These actions will cause your left heel to rise slightly and your left leg to rotate clockwise about the ball of that foot, thereby initiating a step to the left. As your left foot steps, feel the tendency of the pressure on your right foot to move off center, to the inside of that foot. To maintain the distribution of the pressure on the right foot centered, it is necessary for your body to shift exactly the right amount to the right as the left foot steps.

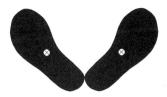

Fig. 7-9. A 50-50 stance, with the heels touching, and each foot is angled at approximately 45 degrees with respect to the starting direction.

Experiment 7-10. Redo Experiment 7-9 in front of a mirror and observe your reflection relative to that of stationary objects behind you. You should see that as you step to the left and keep your weight centered on your right foot, your body will move a small amount to the right.

Stepping While Doing the Form

> **Experiment 7-11.** Slowly do the Taiji form, striving to maintain the pressure distribution on each foot centered as you shift your weight. The more slowly you move, the more your mind will encompass. Each time you shift your weight, feel the pressure distribution centered on the centers of your feet and visualize the line joining their centers. As a stepping leg moves outward, feel the center of the rooted foot, and adjust your center of mass to stay directly over that point.

Note: The above experiments should be practiced until you can readily center the pressure distribution on the center of each foot and stack your center of mass above. Then, recreating those conditions when doing the Taiji form should improve your balance as well as your stability in walking.

Doing Push-Hands

> **Experiment 7-12.** When you do push-hands, strive to maintain the pressure distribution on each foot centered as you shift your weight and turn your body. Each time you shift your weight, feel the conditions of the centers of your feet and the line joining their centers.

Vision

Soft and Hard Vision

Vision and balance are interconnected as evidenced by the need to view the horizon when on a rocking ship to prevent experiencing nausea.

We tend to be habituated to the use of hard vision, which involves fixating the gaze on a small region. Doing so allows us to see detail but requires a certain amount of tension in the musculature of the eyes. Soft vision involves relaxing the musculature of the eyes and processing the entirety of visual sense data. Other than the difference in muscular tension, the main difference between hard and soft vision is how visual sense data is processed.

When you unnecessarily fixate your gaze on one point, you are disregarding sense data of your surroundings and its change with every movement. Increasing your ability to process your surroundings by using soft vision is an invaluable "early warning system" for a loss of balance, which involves an otherwise unnoticed shift of the body.

Most ground animals use soft vision to become aware of the movement of predators or prey. Similarly, animals freeze when they feel they are in danger so they won't be noticed by other animals.

I find that soft vision is quite useful when walking outdoors or driving my car. However, when the need arises, I can shift to hard vision and back.

Experiment 7-13. To practice soft vision, let your eyes float in your eye sockets. Don't become captured by objects. Process all the sense data of the panorama entering your eyes and focused on your retinas. You won't be able to see much detail, but even the slightest shifting movement will be processed.

Experiment 7-14. Using soft vision, attempt to see the white numeral eight composed of the white background between the eight diamonds shown in Figure 7-10.

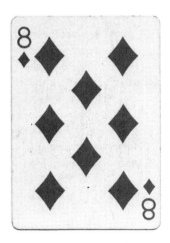

Fig. 7-10. An eight-of-diamonds playing card.

Experiment 7-15. Stand far from a wall or other objects in a room. Raise one leg and move it all the ways you can without losing your balance. Try this experiment two ways: (1) using soft vision and (2) hard vision (look directly at an object). Notice how much better your balance is when you use soft vision.

Conclusion. If you use soft vision when you are practicing balance or simply doing the Taiji movements, you should find that your balance is improved over that of using hard vision.

Retention (Programming Your Subconscious Mind)

Don't worry that you will need to utilize conscious thought continually to retain the beneficial effects of the above experiments. Once you do them sufficiently, their inner knowledge will be emblazoned on your subconscious mind, and you will manifest the benefits automatically.

Other Factors

Awareness of Self and Surroundings

As mentioned, balance requires an awareness and sensitivity of the feet. Most people are not very aware of their feet, which are usually encased in shoes that prohibit movement and sensation. In practicing Taiji, it is necessary to be acutely aware of the placement and angle of each foot and its weight distribution. This awareness then naturally carries over into daily life. Before a fall occurs, there are stages of losing balance. Falling is often preceded by a foot starting to slip or rolling onto its outer edge. The greater the awareness of signals coming from the feet, the earlier corrective action can be taken to restore balance.

Taiji practice involves shifting the weight from one foot to the other and back. Practitioners develop an acute awareness at each moment of the placement and angle of each foot plus the relative weighting of the feet. This feature of Taiji movement cultivates the ability to shift the weight from one foot to the other readily when needed. Thus, when a foot slips or is incorrectly placed, weight can be shifted to the other foot briskly, thus averting a fall.

The mental state practiced in doing Taiji movement carries over to inculcating an awareness of objects in the environment and bodily protective needs. One of my students who is one-hundred one years of age and practices daily, just told me about his experience in falling earlier that day without any appreciable injury. "Even though it only takes a few seconds to reach the floor, it's amazing how much time there is to process everything. As I went down, I was aware of my head, and I made sure that it was tilted forward so it would not hit the floor."

An additional factor in loss of balance is loss of awareness of the motion and positioning of the body relative to the surroundings. Practicing being in the moment is of value in this regard (see "Being in the Moment" in Chapters 9 and 14).

Semicircular Canals

The semicircular canals are interconnected with the hearing apparatus (see Fig. 7-11) but not instrumental in processing sound. Basically, the three canals are mutually perpendicular, aligned in the sagittal, horizontal, and frontal planes. When the body rotates about a vertical axis or tilts forward or sideways, the fluid in the corresponding plane tends to move less than the walls of the canals because of its inertia, causing the fluid to rotate oppositely relative to the rotation of the body. Small hairs arranged on the inside of the canals are then bent, sending sense data to the brain, which results in a perception of how the body is turning. In general, any movement of the body will have components in the three orientations of the canals.

Specific training or awareness of the semicircular canals is, to my knowledge, not something that can consciously be done.

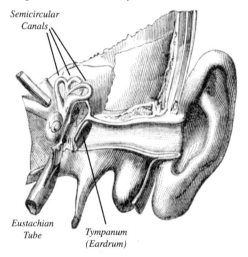

Semicircular Canals

Eustachian Tube

Tympanum (Eardrum)

Fig. 7-11. The hearing apparatus, showing the semicircular canals.[5]

Often, elderly people have sudden, unexplained bouts of dizziness. They are of varying lengths of time and seem to be brought on by changes of position. The medical name given to this condition is *benign paroxysmal positional vertigo*. This condition is thought to be caused by loose crystals in the fluid of the semicircular canals, which give a false sense of movement when none occurs. There are protocols for treating this condition.[6]

---

5. Adapted from Robert Ball, *Wonders of Acoustics* (New York: Charles Scribner & Co., 1870), 237.
6. See https://www.ncbi.nlm.nih.gov/books/NBK458287/.

Chapter 8

An Analysis of "Rooting and Redirecting"

In addition to showing their skill by doing solo movements, push-hands, and self-defense applications, Taiji practitioners also demonstrate "rooting and redirecting." That is, practitioners will stand in a 70-30 stance and pair off with one or more large, strong partners and ask them to push their body or outstretched arm as forcefully as possible. The goal is for practitioners to be so rooted that no movement or loss of balance occurs no matter how hard they are pushed.[1]

Cheng Man-ch'ing was renowned for demonstrating such rooting by standing in the "Ward Off" posture and having one or more partners push his outstretched arm (Fig. 8-1), thereby showing not only rooting but also *peng-jin* skills (*peng* is upward, outward movement or power, and *jin* is refined strength, so *peng jin* is an upward and outward manifestation of refined strength).

How can a small, elderly practitioner withstand a large incoming force without being moved? The analysis of the optimal conditions for rooting requires the use of elementary physics. The quantitative physics derivations will be located in Appendix 2 for reference for those who are interested. A review of the basics of the pertinent vector arithmetic is included in Appendix 1.

Conclusions, intuitive explanations, and experiments are provided in this chapter for those who prefer to skip the physics derivations.

---

1. See video of Chen Xiaowang demonstrating rooting: https://www.youtube.com/watch?v=FtCfUaL-leo.

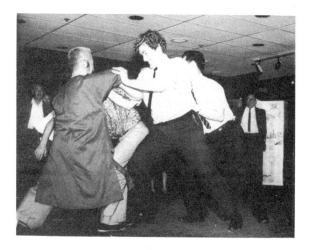

Fig. 8-1. In the above photograph,[2] people are pushing Cheng Man-ch'ing's extended arm. Professor Cheng was renowned for not collapsing his arm and not moving his feet during such demonstrations. The large person in the foreground pushing Professor Cheng's elbow is Patrick Watson (1935–1992).

Conditions for Optimal Stability

The physics analysis (see Appendix 2) reveals the following conditions for optimal stability:

1. Your rear leg must be extended as far back as possible, thereby reducing the angle between the floor and the line along that leg (Fig. 8-2).
2. The body must be positioned such that your partner's point of contact is on the line along your rear leg (Fig. 8-2).
3. Tilting your body forward increases your partner's difficulty in rotating you backward. This condition increases the stabilizing effect of your weight. Interestingly, Professor Cheng's body is not tilted.
4. The more you cause your partner to push you along the line of your rear leg, the greater the frictional force of the floor on your rear foot and the less chance you will slide backward. This condition also aids in reducing your partner's root and traction with the floor.

The question is how you can regulate the direction of the pusher's force to your advantage. To this end, consider next the reaction to the forces exerted by the person pushing. According to Newton's third law, if object *A* exerts a force on object *B* (the action), then *B* exerts an equal-and-opposite force on *A* (the

2. From, *T'ai-Chi Ch'uan, Body and Mind* (New York: Tai Chi Chuan Association, 1968), 32.

reaction). Thus, when your partner exerts a force of magnitude P in a certain direction on you, then you automatically exert a force of magnitude P on him in the opposite direction. If the force of your partner on you has a downward component, your reaction force exerted back on him will automatically have a corresponding upward component. The smaller the angle of the line from the foot to your partner's point of contact, the more you will be rooted (not losing balance or sliding) and the more your partner will be losing balance and traction.

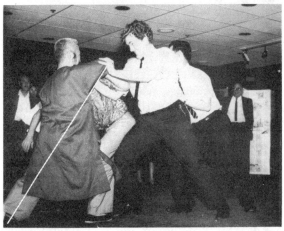

Fig. 8-2. Note that the line drawn from the center of Professor Cheng's rear foot to the point of contact of Patrick Watson is along his rear leg. Note also that Professor Cheng's right arm is pushing Watson's left arm slantingly upward, causing Watson to push Professor Cheng's arm slantingly downward and, thereby, to push himself upward as a reaction to the force he exerts.

So how can you get your partner to push along the line of your rear leg? The answer is that you exert an upward force on your partner, thereby causing him to exert a downward reaction force on you.

Note in Figure 8-2 how Professor Cheng's elbow is lifted, causing Patrick Watson to push partly downward. The combination of downward and forward forces exerted by Watson is then a single resultant force directed toward Professor Cheng's rear foot, thus causing Professor Cheng to be more rooted and less likely to slide backward but lifting Watson, causing him to be less rooted and more likely to tilt and slide backward.

> **Experiment 8-1.** Try pushing the top of a stepladder in the two following ways (or *imagine* doing so). If you push slantingly upward, the ladder will tend to rise, tilt backward, and may even slide backward. Instead, if you push the ladder slantingly downward, it will become immovable.

Internal Aspects

Withstanding another's force without losing your root requires an unobstructed, direct internal path for force exerted on you to pass to the floor. Thus, it is essential to achieve a state of *song*. The contact point of your partner on your body must be totally relaxed and liquid. Moreover, any force you exert on your partner must result from expansion, not contraction.

Experiment 8-2. I learned the following two-person exercise from one of my main teachers, Harvey I. Sober. Min Pai (1934–2004) also showed me a similar exercise at the Shi Zhong school in the early 1970s, when I was too much of a beginner to understand it.

For this experiment, you will need a cooperative partner. Face each other in a 70-30 stance with, say, each person's right foot forward. Then each partner places his or her right hand gently against the chest of the other. Each left hand lightly touches the other's right upper arm.

Alternatively, if one partner is a female, she may choose to place her left forearm against her chest. Her partner's right hand can then touch her forearm instead of her chest and still exert force on her body albeit indirectly. Consequently, her left hand will not contact her partner's right upper arm. That lack of contact is not a problem because in this exercise, the left hand is relatively inactive.

It is essential to attain a state of *song* and that the strength throughout your body and exerted by your pushing hand be expansive. Recognize that any contractive strength in your body is a "handle" that your partner can use to move your center. Similarly, feel how you can utilize such contractive strength in your partner.

As your partner tries to move you with his or her right hand on your chest, make that point of contact a fulcrum; that is, only turn your body about that point, but keep that point stationary. Arrange a lever along a line from your rear foot, through your body, to your partner's hand on your chest, to your right hand on his chest. The lever will not be along a straight line but be resilient and unbending. In this use of leverage, the fulcrum is far from the input end and close to the output end. The lever is, therefore, one that reduces movement but correspondingly multiplies force (see Chapter 5 for a discussion of levers). Do not try to muscle your partner with your right hand.

As your partner exerts force on your chest, sink your weight and expand, thereby unifying your body so that it does not bend under any force that your partner exerts.

(continued on next page)

The magnitude and direction of the force you exert on him with your right hand should be such that the combined effect of that force and the reaction to his force on you is directly to his center and into his weakness. The weakness of your partner's stance is in a direction perpendicular to the line joining the centers of his or her feet and directly to his or her center of mass.

Feel the line of action (it need not be straight) from your rear foot, to your hip joint, to his hand on you (the fulcrum), and to your hand on him. Then arrange the combined effect of his force on you and the reaction to your force on him to be directed to your rear foot. When you feel that your partner is starting to push himself off, then slightly extend your rear leg, causing your partner to increasingly lose balance, with the toes of both feet rising off the floor simultaneously.

The main idea is not to use a lot of force with your hand in breaking your partner's root but rather meet your partner's force in a lever-like response to the force *he exerts on you* with his hand. If this experiment is done properly, your partner will literally break his or her own root, pushing him- or herself increasingly off balance. Of course, the placement of your rear leg, outlined earlier in this chapter, should be observed.

The beauty of this experiment is that it provides immediate feedback for training both partners' alignment, *song*, and expansive strength. With a challenging partner, you will immediately lose your root as soon as one of these elements diminishes.

Chapter 9

Natural Movement

Understanding Natural Movement

What Is Meant by *Natural*.

The word *natural* pertains to *nature*, and a good dictionary will have as many as a dozen definitions of each of these two words. Consider the following definition of *nature*:

> A particular order of existence or of existing things, frequently regarded as in contrast with, or as the subject matter of art. Specif[ically]: a That which is in a natural, as distinct from a developed, ordered, perfected, or man-made state: that which is, or is represented, in its original, untouched condition.[1]

The basic distinction is that *natural* is what existed for approximately 4,000,000,000 years before humans appeared and changed or corrupted it. So we are not here taking the point of view that everything in the world is natural and will not say, for example, that Grand Coulee Dam is as natural as a beaver dam. To do so might be of value in another context—but not here.

Movement in Nature

Movement seen in nature is efficient—if it were not, life forms would be at a great disadvantage. Inefficiency results in wasted time, being noticed by predators, and increased requirements for energy and thermal regulation along with lessened abilities for achieving those requirements. A life-form having these deficiencies would suffer a decreased probability of surviving long enough to reproduce, which would eventually lead to that species's extinction.

In many developed countries in which abundance and safety exist, it is possible to be wasteful of energy, consume unnecessarily, and be unaware of our surroundings safety-wise. But such disregard has health and other consequences.

---

1. *Webster's New International Dictionary of the English Language, 2nd Edition, Unabridged* (Springfield, MA: G. & C. Merriam Co., 1954).

Elements of Natural Movement

Proprioceptive Sense

Proprioceptive sense is the ability to perceive stimuli originating in the tissues of the body resulting from their movement or tension. A large part of learning Taiji involves training the proprioceptive sense to become very keen. Those who teach Taiji know that many beginners have little awareness of their own bodies and move one part thinking that they are moving a totally different part. Or they move the right part but are unaware of how they are moving it. Unless beginners have prior training in dance, sports, or other movement arts, their proprioceptive senses were probably never developed much or were developed at one time and have since atrophied. So studying Taiji can be of great benefit in that respect.

Unified Movement

A basic principle of Taiji is that all movement must be unified, which necessitates feeling all appropriate parts of your body participating as a whole. If you do not know the extent to which each part of your body is involved in a movement—or whether or not it is at rest or moving—it is very hard to manifest unified movement.

Independence of Movement

Practicing independent movement (isolated movement of one part) helps us to become more aware of what part of the body is involved in a particular action and whether it should or should not be involved. How can you know that you are moving in a unified manner if you are unable to move a certain part of your body all the ways it can physiologically move and don't know which parts of the body are initiating each movement? For example, when most people are asked to move a particular region of their spines, they can't do so by using only the muscles around that region and resort to using their pelvises or ribs instead.

By learning to move independently, we can become highly sensitized to frozen or inappropriately used muscle groups, thus providing a tool for directly working on releasing such unnecessary and harmful tension.

Finally, the more able you are to consciously move a particular part of the body independently, the more successful you will be in sending *qi* to that area for healing an injury.

Thus, practicing independent movement can play an important in cultivating proprioceptive sense, ultimately leading to the ability to do unified movement.

Experiment 9-1. Stand in the Jade-Belt posture (Fig. 4-3). Without moving your hands in space, alternately rotate the trunk of your body counterclockwise and clockwise, as a unit. Relax the shoulders and chest and let the inertia of the hands play a large part in keeping them from moving rather than using your eyes and analytical mind to make moment-by-moment adjustments to keep them motionless. Relax your neck and let the inertia of your head keep it from turning as it "floats."

If you have trouble doing this experiment, think about what you do when you are watering your lawn and your neighbor calls to you. Do you turn toward her and spray her? Or does the hose remain in its original direction?

Experiment 9-2. Stand in the Jade-Belt posture (Fig. 4-3) and, as before, alternately rotate the trunk of your body counterclockwise and clockwise as a unit, except this time, slowly and uniformly separate your hands and then bring them together. There should be several cycles of turning of the trunk of the body for each cycle of opening and closing of the arms.

Reasons for Studying Natural Movement

Philosophical

A fundamental Taoist concept in Taiji is achieving naturalness in all action. Another Taoist precept is that an empty cup holds the most; that is, we must strip away our preconceptions and habitual modalities before we can discover the essence of what is natural—our "baggage" obstructs attaining enlightenment.

> Releasing (emptying) as much habitual bodily tension as possible is a precursor to natural movement. Such tension entwines our ways of moving learned by copying inappropriate role models, corrupted early-on by clothing and footwear, and involving subconscious memories of past physical and emotional traumas. We are quite attached to and find it very difficult to change our habitual ways of moving, let alone all manner of other things. To remove a mountain is easy, but to change a man's temperament is harder.[2]
>
> —T. T. Liang (1900–2002)

In recognizing and releasing our physical tensions, we are cultivating the potential ability to release corresponding obstructions in our thinking should we endeavor to do so.

---

2. T. T. Liang, *T'ai Chi Ch'uan for Health and Self-Defense: Philosophy and Practice* (New York: Vintage Books, 1977), 12.

Another philosophical principle that is basic to Taiji is non-action, which means accomplishing a desired action with the minimum effort and movement. Naturalness is akin to non-action because, in nature, wastefulness endangers survival.

In order to recognize and achieve non-action, it is first necessary to release unnecessary tension. Certainly, it is good to get something for free (principle of non-action).

Improvement in Breathing

Many of us do not breathe naturally. Some possible disruptive causes for such an innate and important process are restrictive clothing, the use of tobacco and other inhaled poisonous substances, and the manner in which many of us are birthed. Instead of letting a newly born infant rest and absorb oxygen through the umbilical cord, professionals in maternity wards prematurely sever that cord, forcing an infant to breathe or suffocate. This concept is addressed by Frederick LeBoyer, an obstetrician who has birthed thousands of infants without subjecting them to such unnecessary trauma.[3] This subject is discussed in my *The Tai Chi Book*.[4]

Exercises that emphasize cultivation of contractive strength tend to bind the body and constrict breathing. By contrast, in Taiji and Qigong movement, strength is minimized, enabling breathing to be more natural. Doing only contractive exercise—albeit beneficial—tends to habituate a non-beneficial way of breathing that doing Taiji and other natural activities such as running or swimming can offset.

The question of the advisability of matching breathing with Taiji movements is explored later in this chapter.

A Reduction of "Frozen Tension"

Frozen tension, a term often used by Elaine Summers, refers to maintaining unnecessary muscular tension for long periods of time without an awareness of doing so. That state makes the body unable to move naturally, requires extra energy, restricts needed movement of organs, and cuts off the circulation of blood, lymph, and *qi*.

Sustaining frozen tension is like "driving with one foot on the gas and the other foot on the brakes" and is very hard to recognize because the tensions involved come to feel deceptively natural to us. Such habitual tensions can result from a number of sources, one of which is our "emotional armor," and releasing these unnecessary tensions can make us feel vulnerable.

---

3. Frederick LeBoyer, *Birth Without Violence* (New York: Alfred A. Knopf, 1980).
4. Robert Chuckrow, *The Tai Chi Book* (Wolfeboro, NH: YMAA Publication Center, 1998), 60.

Eventually, frozen tension can become our body identity. It is then possible to do Taiji for quite a while before shedding some of these unnecessary tensions. Learning to free up frozen tension and to move naturally has significant therapeutic value. Then moving naturally, healthfully, and efficiently is exhilarating.

A Reduction of "Sympathetic Tension"

When doing an action requiring strength, we tend to sympathetically tense other muscles that are not appropriate for the job. Such inappropriate usage is a common cause of injury. For example, when doing sit-ups or crunches, some people mercilessly tense their back muscles, thus arching their spines, resulting in chronic back pain. Instead, it is better to extend the lower spine and expand the lower back when doing such exercises.

Injury Prevention

When doing strenuous movement (e.g., lifting a heavy weight), instead of using muscles that are optimal for that action, we tend to use weaker muscles that are physiologically inappropriate. Doing so can cause injury to those weaker muscles.

In doing day-to-day movement, there is also a tendency to avoid use of certain parts of the body, especially when doing so might involve a previously traumatized region. Because we avoid painful actions, parts of the body can become shut off from our awareness. The muscles involved then start to atrophy, causing slow recovery and even further injury. In this regard, learning natural movement and practicing independent movement is very important.

Healing

One of the most efficient ways of healing a part of the body that has been overused or injured is to do relaxed, small movements using the muscles in exactly the region of the injury. It is vital that such movements are done painlessly. When even slight discomfort arises, it is important to suspend the movement causing that discomfort. Then reapproach that movement and do it in a way that does not produce discomfort. In order to take advantage of this powerful method of healing that I learned from Elaine Summers, it is necessary to be able to move each and every part of the body at will.

Developing Expansive Strength

When initially learning to replace contraction by expansion, little expansive strength and its resulting movement are attainable, and the difference between the two types of strength is then difficult to recognize. Lacking the expansive strength to do movement, we then revert to habitual contractive strength, which has a masking effect, making recognition even more difficult.

Similar statements can be made about the importance of attaining the deepest possible state of *song*. We are almost forced to use expansion when we relax contractive strength sufficiently.

Well-timed natural movement allows us to use less strength in general and consequently less contractive strength, thereby promoting the recognition of expansion and its use. Thus, it is important to learn to utilize natural timing of movements of arms, trunk, and legs in relation to the turning of the body to minimize the need for strength of any sort. Experiments along these lines will be provided in this chapter.

Martial

Taijiquan originated as a martial art not primarily based on speed and strength. Because wasteful movement is unnatural, it alerts an opponent and "telegraphs" intention. Thus, moving naturally—in a way that is less likely to be "read" and exploited—provides an advantage over a stronger, faster opponent. Also, moving efficiently, using the smallest possible movements, provides an advantage.

An understanding of natural movement leads to a keen sense of timing necessary to the transfer of mechanical energy to a partner in push hands, which is a precursor for utilizing the optimal timing for defending—or attacking should doing so be required for self-protection.

If you study an art that reduces vulnerability to a trained attacker, you then should be even less vulnerable to becoming injured by inanimate things such as the floor, stairs, or a knife with which you are cutting food. These things are not trying to hurt you, but they can.

Attaining Natural Movement

Cultivating the following issues is a lifelong endeavor. Capturing your movements on video and viewing them in terms of the basic principles has much value in this regard.

Continuity of Movement

Maintaining continuity of motion is a basic principle of Taiji. Yet, it is common to see practitioners freezing the movement of arms and legs at certain points. Often the natural movement of the hands is stopped during stepping. At other times, hands are held in certain positions taught as landmarks to beginners. Two examples are stopping in "Ward Off Left" and freezing the left hand palm up under the right elbow in "Roll Back." Stopping a movement requires force as does starting it again. Thus, a loss of continuity is incompatible with the principle of non-action.

Being in the Moment

Being in the moment is a basic Taiji principle. As soon as you are in the future, you are inattentive to the present, which slips by irrevocably. Then you are in the past, trying to catch up.

Thinking about where a hand is "supposed to be" in the evolution of a movement is an example of not being in the moment and often results in bringing that hand to the expected place prematurely rather than allowing the movement to evolve naturally. It also causes a lack of continuity of motion.

Two examples are reaching the hands to hold a ball in "Ward Off Left" and reaching the left hand to its final position in front of the left shoulder in "Single Whip."

Appropriate Timing

Not recognizing the optimal timing of the turning of the body relative to the swing of the arms for maximizing the transfer of motion to the arms means that extra energy—often muscular tension—is then required, contrary to the principle of non-action.

Natural Stepping

The timing of the stepping relative to the movement of the body is critical and will be covered in the next chapter. Failure to recognize such timing necessitates that muscular action is needed to make up for the lack of what nature provides. Thus, inordinate energy is required for stepping, which is again contrary to the principle of non-action.

Evenness of Rotation of Wrists

In every Taiji movement, the wrists undergo back-and-forth rotations. These rotations have both health and martial aspects. Health-wise, these rotations stretch and release acupuncture meridians, contributing to an increase of *qi*.

Martially, the rotations produce added movement; namely, the wrist contacts the opponent's limb, rotates, and draws the opponent, who then becomes overextended. In both the health and martial cases, when the rotations are done by use of contraction, the functional elements of health and self-defense are lost. When done using expansion, such elements are inculcated.

Shedding Contrived Movement

Instead of artificially causing movement to occur, it is essential to maximally utilize natural factors. Such factors are gravity, momentum, elasticity of tissues when stretched or compressed (internal springs), centrifugal effects of circular motion, and the timing of turning of the trunk of the body relative to the motion of the arms and legs. These factors will be discussed in this and later chapters.

Tools for Studying Natural Movement

Passive and Active Movement

Definition of Passive Movement. *Passive movement* is movement activated by means other than neurological stimulation of muscle fibers or other bodily tissues that would normally produce that movement.

Activators of Passive Movement. The activation for passive movement arises from that of tissues from a different part of the body, restoring force from compression or stretching of tissues, gravity, linear momentum, angular momentum, centrifugal effect, or the action of an outside source such as another person.

Note: Both passive and active movement are equally good when used appropriately, based on conditions.

Examples of Passive Movement. Normally, lifting and lowering your arm involves contraction of muscles in your shoulder, chest, back, etc. But if another person lifts and lowers your arm while your shoulder, chest, and back muscles are in a relaxed state, those muscles lengthen and shorten, not through your own neurological activation but passively, as a result of an action of the muscles of the person doing the lifting.

Another example of passive movement is the hanging exercise of Experiment 7-1, in which the body is lifted by the expansion of the lower abdomen rather than by contraction of the back muscles.

Physics as a Relevant Tool for Studying Natural Movement

Fortunately, physics has extensively analyzed the natural movement of physical systems and studied the conditions under which such movement is produced using minimum external effort. It is of course possible to learn to maximize efficiency without physics, but physics is the appropriate tool for such analysis and for quickly promoting recognition of the essential elements. Therefore, basic physics will be utilized in the analysis that follows.

Note: Because some readers are not proficient in physics, the results will be summarized in plain English and experiments will be provided to facilitate recognition of some important facets of Taiji movement. Just understand the graphics and verbal explanations, and play with the experiments provided. Then you should introduce what you have discovered into your Taiji practice and try your own experiments.

First, some basic physics concepts will be presented. Then passive movement will be analyzed for inanimate objects. Next, passive movement will be discussed for bodily limbs. Finally, self-activated bodily movement will be analyzed to reveal the timing that maximizes movement for a given exertion.

Some Basic Physics Concepts

The Physics Definition of *Stress*

Stress and *strain* are words in everyday usage. Here we will define them in a more scientific way.

Stress. *Stress* is a condition resulting from pressure or opposing forces acting on an object in a manner to deform it. In physics, a number of different types of stress are treated in a qualitative and quantitative manner. Stresses can range from *tensile* (pulling apart), *compression* (crushing), *torsion* (twisting), and *shear* (cutting).

Strain. *Strain* is the object's response to the stress in terms of its amount of deformation.

Tension

When discussing muscular tension, it is important that the scientific meaning of *tension* is understood because ordinary meanings can lead one astray. In physics, the term *tension* refers to a condition arising from the application of outward forces on opposite ends of an object. A good example is a piano string. One end of the string is looped around a stationary hitch pin, embedded in the frame of the piano. The other end is attached to and wound around a tuning pin, which is embedded in a block of wood that is securely fixed to the piano frame. When the tuning pin is rotated in one direction, it increases the tension in the string. The amount of tension is equal to the outward force on *either* end of the string.

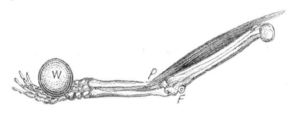

Fig. 9-1. The biceps tendon attaches to point *P* on the radius bone.[5]

The concept of tension can be extended to muscles, but we need to be careful because muscles are animate and have the ability to *produce* force. When muscular action is produced by the contraction of muscle fibers, it results in an outward force exerted on an external object. However, there is

---

5. This figure was reproduced from Edward R. Shaw, *Physics by Experiment* (New York: Maynard, Merrill, & Co., 1897), 28.

still an analogy to a piano string because a bone is connected to a tendon at one end of the muscle involved, and a bone is connected to another tendon at the other end of the muscle involved (see Fig. 9-1).

According to Newton's third law, if object A exerts a force on object B, then B exerts an equal-and-opposite force on A. So by Newton's third law, the amount of tension in the piano-string example above is also the amount of force exerted on either pin by the string.

Newton's third law holds for animate as well as inanimate objects. Therefore, if a muscle exerts a force on a tendon, then the tendon exerts an equal-and-opposite force on the muscle. A similar statement holds for the equality of forces on bones by tendons and that on tendons by bones. Thus, a muscle is under tension when it contracts and causes a force to be exerted on an external object.

Sensing Tension

There is a similarity between our ability to sense tension and a meter used for measuring electrical current (the rate of flow of electrical charge, measured in Amperes; namely, 1 Ampere = 1 Amp = 1 A). Meters have different scales depending on their sensitivity. If small currents are to be measured, the meter must be sensitive enough and have a scale that corresponds to its sensitivity. One meter might have a scale that ranges from 0 to 5 A (Fig. 9-2). Another meter might have a scale that ranges from 0 to 0.5 A, and so on. On the 0–5-Amp scale, 2.5 A will cause a deflection of the needle half way from zero to full scale. One-hundredth of an Ampere might not register at all on the 0–5-A scale and barely on the 0–0.5 Amp scale. But on a meter having a scale that ranges from 0 to 0–0.05-A (Fig. 9-3), the needle will move to one fifth of full scale.

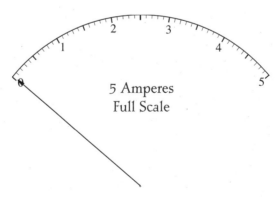

5 Amperes
Full Scale

Fig. 9-2. A current of 0.01 Amps applied to an ammeter with a full-scale deflection of 5 Amps.

As humans, our range of sensory ability is analogous to that of the meters just discussed. If we are providing a large stimulus to our nervous system by our own tension, then we will be less sensitive to our use of strength and our contriving movement rather than letting it occur by natural means. So not relaxing tension sufficiently will reduce progress in Taiji.

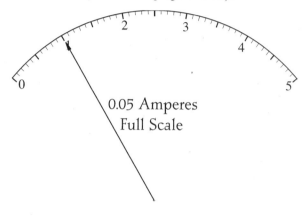

Fig. 9-3. A current of 0.01 Amps applied to an ammeter with a full-scale deflection of 0.05 Amps.

Elasticity

Elasticity is the property of a medium that results in it resuming its original configuration when released after being distorted (compressed, stretched, or twisted). The force that the medium exerts back on the agent that distorts it is called a *restoring force*. Examples of elastic substances are rubber, steel, glass, and some plastics. Of course, bodily tissues have elasticity, and the goal is to recognize and utilize that feature in Taiji movement.

Hooke's Law

Hooke's law pertains to an elastic medium that is displaced from its equilibrium condition (*equilibrium* means that all forces are balanced). Hooke's law states that the restoring force F is proportional and opposite to the displacement x from equilibrium.

$$F = -kx$$

The negative sign before the proportionality constant k indicates that the restoring force F is opposite to the displacement x. The larger the k, the greater the restoring force exerted by the object. Thus, k is referred to as the *stiffness constant*.

As an example of Hooke's law, consider a coil spring, hung from the ceiling (Fig. 9-4). If a weight w is added to the bottom of the spring, the spring will stretch by a certain amount x. If instead, $2w$ is added, then the spring will stretch by $2x$. Then if $3w$ is added, the spring will stretch by $3x$, and so on. That is, the stretch of the spring is proportional to the force stretching it. Alternatively stated, the spring's restoring force increases proportionally to the amount it is stretched.

Of course, there is a limit to how much weight can be added for a proportional stretch of the spring. Moreover, if sufficient weight is added, the spring will break.

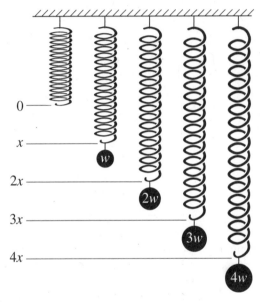

Fig. 9-4. Five states of a hanging spring are shown. The stretch of the spring is proportional to the amount of added weight.

Applying Hooke's law to the case of bodily tissues, first consider the case in which bodily tissues lengthen, either actively or passively. As the tissues lengthen, their natural elasticity creates increasing tension proportional to the degree of the excursion from the equilibrium condition.

Elasticity of Bodily Tissues

According to Hooke's law, as any part of the body (arm, leg, trunk, etc.) lengthens or bends away from its neutral position, the natural elasticity of the stretched tissues (muscles, fascia, skin, blood vessels, nerves, tendons, etc.) creates an increasing restoring tension. At a certain degree of lengthening of the tissues, their elastic restoring force can now become a significant factor. That effect can be felt more when doing stretching by extension than by contraction.

Compressional Stress

We have discussed the elasticity and stress involved in the elongation of an object such as a spring. There is, however, another kind of stress called *compressional stress*, which occurs not only in springs, which are inanimate, but in living tissues such as those surrounding the hip, shoulder, and knee joints. Thus, compressed tissues have spring-like effects. Such an effect is discussed in conjunction with Taiji movements such as "Single Whip" later in this chapter.

Consider what might occur if an opponent exerts a large force on you when your body is in a state of unified expansion. If it is true that expansion is a result of a modified state of water, then the effect of the opponent's force is to pressurize that water. Water has a compressional property that is analogous to that of a very large spring constant k; that is, a large pressure produces only a small reduction in volume. The effect of pressurized water in bodily tissues, when electrified to become a gel, can then be protective against an incoming strike. This idea is consistent with the ability of high-level Taiji and Qigong masters to take a powerful punch comfortably.

"Swinging," an element of the training of such a skill, is treated in Chapter 11. Such training involves repeated tapping of the body by the arms and hands. It is known that tapping the body results in an automatic, local electrical response. That electricity may then activate water in the tissues to become protective. With repeated training, an almost immediate protective response to an incoming force occurs.

Whereas practicing expansion inculcates an expansive bodily tone that persists even when asleep, practicing repetitive tapping intensifies this tone so that when the body is struck—even lightly—the expansive response is immediate.

The ability of high-level masters in "springing" out an opponent or partner with little or no appreciable outward movement may also be associated with the high compressibility of water.[6]

Animate and Inanimate Natural Movement

Naturally Occurring Compression and Tension in "Single Whip"

The "Single Whip" movement occurs six times in the Cheng Man-ch'ing short form and eleven times in the Yang long form. It is evidently a movement whose elements are important. Other movements that are similar to "Single Whip" are the "Four Corners." In these movements, there is an opening and closing of the hip joints (*kua*) beyond that in most other movements.

---

6. See, for example, https://www.youtube.com/watch?v=XSnUDkCQ0WU.

The "Single Whip" starts (say from the 70-30 position of "Push") by sitting back 100 percent onto the rear (left) leg, which is turned in 45 degrees. Then the body turns 90 degrees to the left (the feet are now turned 45 degrees inward), thereby compressing the tissues of the left hip joint and stretching the musculature in the back. Releasing this stored spring energy causes the body to open and shift to the right leg, which is now turned in 45 degrees. Now the tissues of the right hip joint become compressed as the body turns to the right as a result of its turning momentum. Releasing this stored spring energy causes the body to open into its final position.

Utilizing the turning of the body by releasing compressed and stretched springs is achieved "free of charge." The result is that the body shifts, turns, and steps seamlessly and naturally. Without utilization of spring action, it is necessary to "throw" the body, which is awkward and negatively affects balance and the continuity of the movement.

Baguazhang, another internal art, which involves circular motion while walking in a circle, routinely utilizes spring energy similar to that just described in "Single Whip." Baguazhang movements begin with *kobu* (turning the body and empty foot inward) and *beibu* (opening and stepping using the spring energy of the *kua*).

Experiment 9-3. Stand with feet parallel and a comfortable distance apart. Extend one arm forward at mid-chest level and relax the arm as much as possible. Feel the neutral orientation of your wrist and forearm rotation-wise. Slowly rotate your wrist and forearm in one direction (say, clockwise). Feel the resistance build proportionally to the degree of rotation. Then slowly let the wrist and forearm return to the neutral orientation. Repeat in the other direction.

Experiment 9-4. Stand with arms in the "Jade-Belt" orientation (see Fig. 4-3), with everything as relaxed as possible. Then slowly bring the arms apart, and feel the upper arms, shoulders, and chest. Notice how the elasticity in the tissues of those regions of the body increase in resistance as the arms open even though they are not actively tensing.

Note: It is important when doing the kind of movement described in the above two exercises that you recognize what Sam Chin Fan-siong called your "limit of strength." That is, at a certain point, expansive strength is insufficient to overcome the elastic restoring force of the displaced tissues, and there is then a tendency to use contraction to exceed that limit.

Twisting the Body

Twisting means that one part of the body (say, the chest) is turning a different amount than another part (say, the pelvis). In Taiji movement, the trunk of the body does not actively twist. The basic idea is that if twisting occurs, the body is not unified or strong, and the power is then much less than if the body is turning as a unit.

Active Versus Passive Twisting

Active twisting occurs when the top parts of the body (arms, shoulders, chest) turn by means of intention and muscular contraction beyond the amount that the lower body (legs and pelvis) turns, thereby twisting the spine and trunk of the body. Active twisting is a defect; it is weak and inconsistent with unified movement, which results when expansion permeates every part of the body.

To understand passive twisting, it is important to realize that nothing is totally rigid—not even steel. When my garage was being built, a truck arrived with an I-beam on top. I easily saw its ends were lower than its middle. I said to the truck driver, "This I-beam is not straight!" He replied, "It's not straight now but it will be when the upper story is added." And after the upper story was completed, I sighted along the beam and it was perfectly straight.

Of course, even when unified, the body is not totally rigid, and the trunk can twist very slightly. When, for example, the body turns to the right and the legs and hips stop, the upper body will continue to turn slightly and there will be twisting due to its residual rotational momentum. Such natural twisting is not active but occurs passively because the body is not rigid.

"Rollback and Press" can be used to illustrate the distinction between active and passive twisting. Active twisting occurs when the pelvis reaches its limit of turning, and then the shoulders continue to turn by muscular action, thereby twisting the spine and trunk of the body.

Passive twisting occurs when the pelvis reaches its limit of turning, and the rotational momentum results in the upper body continuing to turn slightly until a counterforce resulting from the elasticity of the tissues brings the turning to a stop.

Condensing and Expanding

Sam Chin Fan-siong, frequently emphasized what he called *condensing and expanding*. Whereas Chinese was Chin's native language, he used English words with much thought, care, and precision. Chin writes about his system in his book on I Liq Chuan, translated as *mind, body self-defense*.[7]

By the word *condensing*, Chin meant that whereas the *yang* part of each movement involves an expansion of strength originating from the centers of

---

7. Sam F.S. Chin, *I Liq Chuan: Martial Art of Awareness* (Mount Kisco, NY: Chin Family I Liq Chuan Association, 2006).

the feet, the *yin* part of each movement involves a controlled *release* of expansion. That is, condensing involves decreasing—but not losing—the state of expansion. This release allows the natural elasticity of the tissues to produce an inward movement passively.

In physics and chemistry, the term *condensing* applies to a system for which the motion of the molecules decreases. For a confined gas, this slowdown results in the molecules hitting the walls of the container (a) with less force and (b) less frequently. Each of these factors causes a decrease in pressure on the walls of the container enclosing the gas. So characterizing the reduction of bodily expansion by using the word *condensing* is therefore apt.

Once you have become proficient in expanding, you can start to work on condensing. The inward and downward (*yin*) parts of each movement are facilitated by condensing, and the upward and outward (*yang*) parts of each movement are facilitated by expansion. Thus, condensing and expanding alternate when doing Taiji movement.

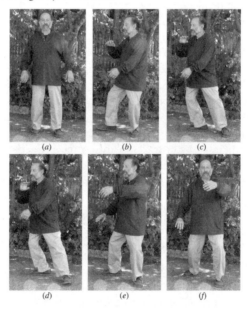

Fig. 9-5. The author moving from the "Beginning" Taiji posture to "Ward Off Left."

For example, consider the condensing and expanding that might occur in moving from the "Beginning" posture to "Ward Off Left." At the final part of "Beginning," your elbows are rotated slightly forward, your palms face the rear, and your hands are outside and slightly forward of your thighs (Fig. 9-5a). As you shift your weight 100 percent to the left foot and turn to the right, your right arm simultaneously begins rising and becomes expanded, and your left arm moves with the body (Fig. 9-5b). As you shift your weight to your right foot, holding a "ball" with your right hand on top, the expansion of your right arm decreases and that of your left arm increases as it continues its movement (Fig. 9-5c). As you sink into the right foot to step with the left foot, the expansion of the insides of the thighs should also accompany and facilitate the opening of the hip joints (Fig. 9-5d). At the same time, your left arm is already rising by means of expansion and steadily continues its upward, outward, circular motion as you step, turn slightly, and start to shift (Fig. 9-5e). After you shift 70 percent onto the left leg, you continue turning to finish the movement (Fig. 9-5f). By now, your left arm is expanded upward and outward, and your right arm has lowered to the same position as it was after the "Beginning" posture.

Condensing Versus Contracting

The expression *contracting and expanding* is sometimes used to characterize the alternation from *yin* to *yang* throughout the form. Actually, contracting and expanding are *both yang*; contracting is actively pulling inward by using muscular tension. By comparison, *condensing* implies a decrease in outward pressure—not anything pulling inward as in the case of contraction. So condensing is *yin*.

Condensing and Expanding for "Receiving Energy"

Professor Cheng Man-ch'ing described "attracting" an opponent's powerful force and then discharging it, which he called "receiving energy."[8] He said that such an ability was the highest level of Taiji and is different from using "force against force."[9]

One of my major teachers, Harvey I. Sober, spoke about a similar concept of absorbing an opponent's energy and then "spitting" it out.

For receiving energy to work, the timing and power of the condensing and expanding of the body must be absolutely perfect. In one class, Professor Cheng let a student punch him a few times in his abdomen with full power. The student stood a distance from Cheng and briskly stepped forward to punch, thus adding the full momentum of his body. I carefully watched Professor Cheng and saw that just before the punch landed, his abdomen slightly receded and then visibly expanded as the punch landed. Each time the punch hit, it made a loud sound. Professor Cheng was obviously unharmed.

---

8. Cheng Man-ch'ing, *Tai Chi Chuan: A Simplified Method of Calisthenics for Health and Self Defense* (Berkeley, CA: North Atlantic Books, 1985), 10.

9. Cheng Man-ch'ing, *Tai Chi Chuan*, 124–5.

Inner Washing

Harvey Sober talked about the concept of inner washing. The movements of Taiji and Qigong have a natural ebb and flow. As the external movement involves backward and forward, down and up, and closing and opening, there are corresponding internal changes. These changes serve to move organs, glands, and other tissues in a manner that beneficially stimulates *qi*, cellular absorption of oxygen and nutrients, and elimination of metabolic wastes. It also aids in the redistribution of material within the cells.

These processes are analogous to washing clothes in a washing machine. Agitation and rinsing enable movement of surfactants into clothing and dirt out. Doing Taiji and Qigong movements with such recognition enhances these effects. Moreover, condensing and expanding at appropriate parts of each movement further enhance cellular cleansing.

The movements "Rollback and Press" and "Withdraw and Push" are especially useful in practicing inner washing because they involve only shifting and turning but no stepping.

Cerebrospinal Flow

The cerebrospinal flow is a phenomenon discovered in the mid-1700s and recognized and studied by modern medicine.[10] Utilized in certain massage modalities, it involves an upward expansion of the spinal fluid to the brain and then a downward release of this fluid. The cycle repeats about every six seconds and can be readily felt when quietly sitting or standing. It is experienced as a swelling of the head, followed by its release.

I have found that when doing the Taiji form, I tend to automatically synchronize some of the forward and backward movements with the cerebrospinal flow.

The movements in the sequence "Ward Off Right," "Roll Back," "Withdraw and Push" naturally lend themselves to cultivating such a synchronization because of their back-and-forth movement without any stepping. The forward movement corresponds to the cerebrospinal expansion, and the backward movement corresponds to the cerebrospinal condensation.

On Matching Breathing with Taiji Movements

Some Taiji teachers emphasize inhaling at the end of a movement, and others emphasize exhaling. Also, some teachers emphasize natural breathing, and others—especially those with martial backgrounds—emphasize reverse breathing.

To my knowledge, Professor Cheng did not provide us with any rule about how or when to breathe. The only thing I ever heard him say in that regard pertained to the "Beginning" movement. He said, "As the arms rise, you're

---

10. https://en.wikipedia.org.

breathing in, and as they descend, you're breathing out. *The rest takes care of itself.*" (Author's emphasis.)

When I was a beginner in Taiji, someone knowledgeable about martial arts asked me, "Are you being taught the breathing?" When I said that I wasn't, his response was, "You are not getting the true teaching."

Breathing *was* emphasized and taught by my successive teachers. One teacher taught inhaling at the end of a movement, which I then practiced. Later teachers taught exhaling at the end of a movement, and I practiced doing that. Eventually, I understood the physiology of reverse breathing, which I practiced for years, exhaling at the end of each movement.

I no longer intentionally match breathing to the movements. That does not mean that I don't do a particular modality of breathing. I tend to automatically do a gentle form of reverse breathing when doing the form but have no rule about when I should be inhaling or exhaling. Instead, I let the timing aspect of my breathing respond to the needs of the moment. The following is my reasoning.

It is natural to inhale when the arms rise and open outward, and it is natural to exhale when they lower and close inward. When the arms rise and open, the ribs and lower abdomen tend to expand, bringing in air. When the arms lower and close, the ribs and lower abdomen naturally tend to move inward, consistent with exhaling.

In the short form and especially the long form, some of the final postures are very open, but some are closed. For example, "White Crane," "Single Whip," "Diagonal Flying," "Parting the Wild Horse's Mane," and "Fan through the Back" all end in a very open posture consistent with an inhalation. On the other hand, "Fist under Elbow," "Needle a Sea Bottom," and "Step Up to the Seven Stars" all end in a closed posture consistent with an exhalation. So a one-size-fits-all rule about always inhaling or exhaling at the end of a posture leads to a physiological contradiction.

Breathing is one of the most important bodily functions. We can go without food for many weeks, without water for maybe a few days, but without air for only a few minutes.

Humans have evolved from simpler life forms for about 4,000,000,000 years. After so long, it would seem that our bodies would be quite able to know when to inhale or exhale. So when I do the form, even though I do reverse breathing, I leave it up to nature when to inhale, exhale, or naturally suspend breathing.

Regularly practicing inhaling or exhaling at the end of a movement adversely overrides the natural tendency of the body to fulfill its moment-by-moment needs and should be put aside. The result of letting the breathing take care of itself is that inhalations, exhalations, and their depth all occur naturally, without any preconceived idea or intervention.

Not matching breathing in the meditative movement of the Yang and Cheng Man-ch'ing styles does not preclude doing so in styles involving alternation of meditative and explosive movement such as in Chen style. Moreover, doing breathing exercises and experimenting with all manner of breathing are of great value.[11]

Understanding the Natural Swing of Our Limbs

We next explore the various passive-movement modalities of the arms and legs. In order to understand the free motion of our limbs, which consist of bones and soft tissue, we will first consider an inanimate system that can swing analogously. We will first analyze the motion of a simple pendulum and then different ways that a frictionlessly pivoted rod can swing, either freely or resulting from various movements of the pivot. The results will aid in understanding the various passive-movement modalities of the arms and legs.

Simple Pendulum (Modality 1)

A simple pendulum can be easily constructed from a length of string. One end of the string is looped around a stationary pivot, and a weight is attached to the other end (Fig. 9-6a). The weight can be displaced to the side so the string makes an angle θ_i with the vertical. Then the weight is released and swings back and forth (Fig. 9-6b and c). The number of complete swings per second is called the *frequency f*. It turns out that the frequency does not depend on the mass but only on the length of the string; the longer the string, the longer the frequency.

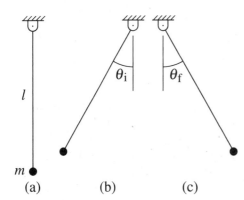

Fig. 9-6. (a) An ordinary pendulum consisting of a weight (called a *bob*) attached to a length *l* of string looped around a pivot, hanging at rest. (b) The bob is displaced so that the string makes an initial angle θ_i with the vertical and then released. (c) It swings to its highest level on the other side, making a final angle θ_f with the vertical, and continues swinging back and forth with decreasing amplitude due to friction.

If there were no friction, gravity would be the only force doing work, mechanical energy would be conserved, and θ_f would equal θ_i. But the

---

11. For some breathing experiments, see Robert Chuckrow, *Tai Chi Dynamics* (Wolfeboro, NH: YMAA Publication Center, 2008), 21–22.

dissipative effects of friction of the air and of the pivot cause the amplitude of motion to decrease, and the bob will eventually come to rest.

Note: We will explore the natural swing of arms and legs in the following examples. Because elementary physics is the appropriate tool for such explorations, derivations simulating limbs by pivoted rods are included in Appendix 3 for reference for those who are interested in the physics. We will then provide conclusions, intuitive explanations, and experiments in this chapter for those who prefer to skip the physics.

Swing of a Frictionlessly Pivoted Rod When Displaced and Released (Modality 2)

We next consider a rod hanging from a frictionless pivot, displaced at an angle θ_i and then released (Fig. 9-7 a). The motion of the rod should approximate that of a relaxed arm hanging from a shoulder after being similarly displaced and then released. As with the simple pendulum, the rod swings to its highest level on the other side (Fig. 9-7 b), making a final angle θ_f with the vertical, and continues swinging back and forth with decreasing amplitude due to friction.

As with the simple pendulum, for the first swing, with θ_f approximately equal to θ_i, the amplitude of motion decreases, and the rod eventually comes to rest.

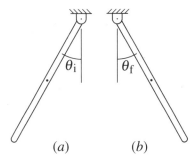

(a)   (b)

Fig. 9-7. A physical pendulum, consisting of a rod of length l, mass m, hanging from a frictionless, stationary pivot. (a) The rod is displaced so that it makes an initial angle θ_i with the vertical. (b) The rod swings to its highest level on the other side, making a final angle θ_f with the vertical.

> **Experiment 9-5.** In a standing position, let your arm hang. Feel its weight, and release as much tension in your arm and shoulder as possible. Then, without moving your shoulder, have somebody lift your arm forward and release it. Note how your arm swings backward and then forward, nearly at the same height from which it started. Then it swings back and forth with decreasing amplitude until it comes to rest.

Observe how becoming more relaxed increases the number of swings before your arm comes to rest.

Horizontally Moving Rod After the Pivot Is Suddenly Fixed (Modality 3)

We are next interested in the swing of a hanging rod when the pivot is moving forward (or backward) and then stops (see Appendix 3 for a quantitative treatment of this modality).

Conclusion. At the moment that the pivot stops, the rod swings toward the direction that the pivot was originally moving and rises an appreciable amount before stopping and swinging back.

Intuitive explanation. When the pivot of the hanging rod is suddenly stopped, the top of the rod must also come to a stop. But all of the other particles of the rod have movement, which tends to continue. So the resulting motion of the rod is rotational about the pivot. However, the pull of gravity slows down the upward rotation until the rod momentarily stops and then swings backward.

> **Experiment 9-6.** Let your arm loosely hang from your shoulder while moving your shoulder forward. Then suddenly stop your shoulder's movement. Note how your arm continues to move forward. Then it will swing back and forth with decreasing amplitude until it comes to a stop.

Swing of a Frictionlessly Pivoted, Hanging Rod When the Pivot Is Then Accelerated Horizontally (Modality 4)

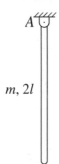

A

$m, 2l$

Fig. 9-8. A rod of length mass m, $2l$, motionlessly hanging from a frictionless pivot (point A). The pivot is then accelerated to the right.

Again consider a rod motionlessly hanging from a frictionless pivot, when the pivot is suddenly accelerated (see Appendix 3 for a quantitative treatment of this modality). The motion of the rod should approximate that of a relaxed arm hanging from a shoulder similarly accelerated (Fig. 9-8).

Conclusion. When the pivot of the rod (at its top) is accelerated to the right by a, the bottom of the rod is suddenly accelerated in the opposite direction (to the *left*) by $a/2$.

Intuitive explanation. When the pivot of the hanging rod is suddenly moved to the right, the top of the rod must also move to the right. But all of the other particles of the rod have inertia, which results in their tending to lag behind. So the resulting motion of the rod is a backward rotation about the pivot.

Experiment 9-7. Let your arm hang loosely from your shoulder. Then accelerate your shoulder forward by turning your body. Note how your arm initially swings backward.

Experiment 9-8. Watch people walk. Observe that as the rear knee starts to move forward and the rear foot becomes airborne, the lower leg momentarily swings backward.

Experiment 9-9. Try doing "Ward Off Left," starting at the end of the "Beginning" posture facing north (the starting direction is arbitrarily defined to be north). See how the modalities just derived apply as follows.

As you shift your weight 100 percent onto your left leg and turn your body clockwise, your left shoulder also turns clockwise, creating an eastward component of motion of your left shoulder. Note how your left arm initially swings westward (modality 4). Then, as you shift to the right, your shoulder moves farther to the right, causing your left arm to swing even more to the left (modality 4). That arm will now make a sizable angle with the vertical. When you stop shifting and step toward the starting direction with your left foot, your left arm will swing and rise to at least the same angle as on the other side (modalities 2 and 3). Finally, as you shift your weight to 70 percent on the left leg, turn, and stop, your left arm will rise (modality 4). Of course, at this point, you will need some expansive strength to bring your left arm to its final height at sternum level.

Note: The results of the prior modalities (2, 3, and 4) and their accompanying Experiments will help in understanding leg motion in the next chapter on "stepping like a cat" and the relationship of the turning of the body and the circular motion of the arms in the chapter after that on periodic motion. Those modalities are (2) the swing of a pivoted rod when displaced and released; (3) the swing of a pivoted, hanging, horizontally moving rod after the pivot is suddenly fixed; and (4) the swing of a pivoted, hanging rod when the pivot is horizontally accelerated. All of these modalities come into play when an outside agent adds motion efficiently to a vibrating system.

Potential and Kinetic Energy

When you rub two objects together, the work you perform is transformed into thermal energy. Equivalently said, the objects experience a rise in temperature. The work you performed increased the random motion of the molecules but not the motion of the object as a whole. However, when you throw something, the work you do goes into increasing *ordered* motion of all of the molecules of the object—not randomly but all of them having the same increase of motion in the same direction. Both of these increases in motion—random and uniform—are said to correspond to an increase in *kinetic energy* (KE) (energy of motion).

Now, if you slowly lift an object through a vertical distance, the work you do against gravity does not go into KE (either thermal energy or an increase in motion of the object as a whole). However, the work you did is not lost but is "potentially available." Here is why: if the object were dropped, gravity would then do the same amount of work as you originally expended in lifting it, and the motion of the object would have increased by the same amount as if you did that work by accelerating the object the same amount as that done by gravity.

The above situation of lifting and then dropping the object is described by saying that when lifting the object, we increased its *potential energy* (PE), and when dropping it, the decrease in PE went into an equal increase in *kinetic energy* (KE).

Similarly, when you stretch or compress a spring or any elastic medium, the work done is transformed into PE, which can then become KE (e.g., a bow and arrow).

The main idea is to recognize that the energy you expend in lifting an arm or leg or squeezing or stretching a part of the body is not necessarily lost. If you can relax contractive tension sufficiently and become aware of subtleties, you can then do a lot of movement "free of charge."

Chapter 10

Stepping Like a Cat[1]

Taiji Stepping

In the Taiji Classics, Wu Yu-hsiang says, "When changing position, you should move like a cat."[2] That admonition implies that you should step naturally, as a cat would. When stalking a bird or a mouse, a cat does not commit any weight onto a stepping paw before it is already touching the ground. Committing its weight prematurely would produce a discontinuity in motion that alerts its prey (in the footnote below, watch a youtube.com video of a jaguar stalking and seizing a crocodile).[3] Moreover, a cat would not stiffen its joints while walking.

However, when stepping, some Taiji practitioners lift and move their legs stiffly as rigid units instead of releasing their knee joints and allowing their lower legs to swing freely. Also, some practitioners literally fall onto a stepping foot, with the floor preventing a complete fall.

Stepping in this manner is unnatural, breaks the balance and continuity of *yin* and *yang*, and increases vulnerability to falling in daily life. It is also martially incorrect because an opponent can easily become alerted by the discontinuity and take advantage of options such as sweeping the stepping foot just as it hits the ground. The balance of *yin* and *yang* and their continuity of mutual exchange are essential to Taiji. Thus, the stepping foot, which is *yang* (active, upward, outward), must continuously evolve into *yin* (earthy, supportive, inactive) as it blends with the ground.

---

1. Much of the material of this chapter was originally published as an article: Robert Chuckrow, "Stepping Like a Cat," *Qi: The Journal of Traditional Eastern Health & Fitness.* 24, no. 3 (Autumn, 2014).

2. Waysun Liao, *T'ai-Chi Classics* (Boston: Shambhala, 2000), 122.

3. https://www.youtube.com/watch?v=DBNYwxDZ_pA.

Yin and Yang

The concept of *yin* and *yang* is basic to the art of Taiji. In fact, the *yin-yang* symbol (Fig. 10-1) and the art are both called *Taiji*. Thus, it is essential to adhere to the principles expressed by the *yin-yang* symbol in doing Taiji movement.

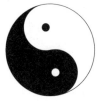

Fig. 10-1. The Taiji symbol, which portrays the balance of *yin* and *yang* and their continuous cyclic evolution. The dark part is *yin*, and the light part is *yang*.

The Taiji symbol portrays the balance and cyclic interchange of *yin* and *yang*. We see circularity, continuity, and balance. Note that in the Taiji symbol, *yin* and *yang* continuously alternate, one into the other, as do night and day. When *yang* becomes full, it starts to become *yin*, and vice versa.

Weight Transfer

The graphs below display the correct and the incorrect build-up of force on the ground during stepping into a 70-30 stance (Figs. 10-2 and 10-3, respectively). In these graphs, t_i and t_p are the times for the weight on the stepping foot to stabilize at 7 percent for proper and improper stepping, respectively.

In proper stepping (Fig. 10-2), the foot blends with the ground, and the force builds up uniformly to 70 percent. In improper stepping (Fig. 10-3), instead of the foot blending with the ground (as in Fig. 10-2), the force builds up very quickly to a level above 70 percent because of the momentum of the moving (actually falling!) body while stepping. Next, the practitioner executes a series of successively decreasing over-corrections.

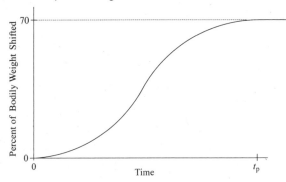

Fig. 10-2. A graph of force of the practitioner's stepping foot on the ground versus time for proper stepping. Note that the force builds up smoothly as does *yang* into *yin* in the Taiji symbol (Fig. 10-1).

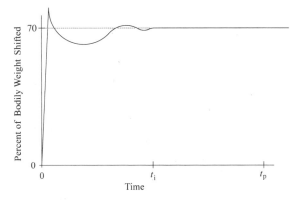

Fig. 10-3. A graph of force of the practitioner's stepping foot on the ground versus time for improper stepping.

Weight Transfer when Sitting Down

The above principles can be extended to sitting down on a chair, something we do many times a day. Most people walk up to a chair, turn, and literally fall into the chair. Instead, true Taiji practitioners lower themselves slowly and first contact the chair without any commitment. Then, they mindfully transfer weight until it is safe to commit it fully.

The problem with falling into the chair is that the chair might have been moved or may slide when you make contact. I know someone who seriously injured her spine when attempting to sit on a chair she thought was there but was not. A few years ago, I was working on two computers at the same time (multitasking). I left one computer and went to sit down on the other chair, unaware that someone had removed it. When I lowered myself and felt nothing, I safely rose and thanked Taiji for not being injured or even having fallen.

Difficulties in Stepping Like a Cat

Strength and Range of Movement of Legs

In order to "step like a cat," it is necessary that the stepping foot be low enough to blend with the ground so continuously that there is almost no perception of the foot contacting the ground. That condition requires the rooted leg to have (a) sufficient strength to stably support the full weight of the body and (b) a sufficient range of motion to bend enough for the stepping foot to easily reach the ground without losing stability.

Alignment

Proper alignment of the knee, ankle, and arch is essential. Knee, ankle, and arch alignment is discussed in my book *Tai Chi Walking*[4] and my Internet article.[5] When the rooted knee pronates (caves inward), stability is adversely affected, and the rooted leg becomes weak and even painful when bent to the required degree. Four problems can then arise: (1) The wear and tear of habitual repetition can eventually take its toll in degeneration of the knee joint. (2) The knee and ankle are off-center, which greatly increases the probability of a sudden injury such as a sprain. (3) The arch becomes collapsed, which places inordinate pressure on the first metatarsal and negates the shock-absorbing function of the arch. (4) The ability to exert force on an external object or another person is limited because the reaction[6] to the exerted force becomes damaging to the incorrectly aligned joints. Centering the pressure distribution on the center of a foot (discussed in Chapter 7) is a large factor in attaining optimal foot/ankle/knee alignment.

Balance

When balance is off, it is almost impossible to step like a cat. Poor balance often results from insufficient leg strength, failure to center the pressure distribution on the the center of each foot, and fixating rather than softening the vision (see Chapter 7). Feeling the center of mass of the body directly above the center of the weighted leg is also important.

Range of Opening of the Hip Joints

Much of the stepping in Taiji movement—especially in the Cheng Man-ch'ing short form—involves opening the thigh bones by 90 degrees and in some cases 135 degrees. When the corresponding muscles lack sufficient range for opening the hip joints sufficiently, there is a tendency to pronate the rooted knee (cave that knee inward) to make up for that lack. Aside from the physiological price paid for that incorrect alignment, the result can also be awkward stepping.

Sinking the Weight (*Song*)

Truly sinking the weight onto one leg requires releasing the thigh muscles totally, resulting in their being stretched to their limit by the weight of the body. If these muscles are not able to withstand that kind of stress, they contract to protect themselves from injury. In that case, achieving *song* is

---

4. Robert Chuckrow, *Tai Chi Walking* (Wolfeboro, NH: YMAA Publication Center, 2002), 17–23.

5. https://www.chuckrowtaichi.com/Alignment.html.

6. Newton's third law of motion can be stated, "If *A* exerts a force on *B*, then *B* exerts an equal-and-opposite force on *A*." *A*'s force can be thought of as the action, and *B*'s force can be thought of as the reaction.

difficult, and stepping is awkward. Regular practice in which such contraction is gradually lessened results in eventual strengthening and lengthening of the leg muscles. Here, correct alignment is crucial because sinking into an incorrectly aligned leg can result in chronic or acute injury.

Order of Stepping: Heel First, Toe First, or Whole Foot?

Figure 10-4 shows the swing of the foot about the hip joint in natural stepping. In stepping forward (position *c*), the lowest point is the heel, whereas in stepping backward (position *a*), the lowest point is the toe. Therefore, in stepping forward, it is natural to contact the ground with the heel first, and in stepping backward, it is natural to contact the ground with the toe first.

Note that in stepping forward or backward, the leg arcs upward and raises the foot. Thus, it is necessary that the rooted leg is sufficiently bent; otherwise the stepping foot will not reach the ground, and the step will involve "falling" onto that foot. An evident reason that beginners step forward toe-first is that it is hard for them to sink low enough for the heel of a stepping foot to touch first, so they reach with their toes.

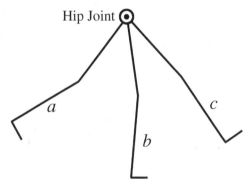

Fig. 10-4. Swing of the leg during stepping forward or backward. The hip joint is the point about which there is a swiveling action.

Stepping to the Side

It is logical from the prior discussion that, when stepping to the side, neither the toe nor heel touch first—all the parts of the sole of the foot that normally contact the floor in correct standing alignment should touch at the same time (Figs. 10-5 and 10-6). Such an action involves a hinge-like motion of the hip joint and requires bending at the ankle to keep the foot from tilting or caving in at the arch.

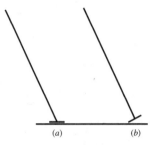

(a)   (b)

Fig. 10-5. When stepping to the side, the sole of the foot should be parallel to the ground as in (a). The foot should not be angled to the ground as in (b).

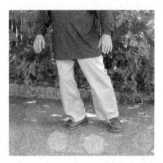

Fig. 10-6. The correct way for the foot to initially contact the ground when stepping to the side—with the sole of the foot parallel to the ground.[7]

Why should stepping to the side involve the whole foot touching the ground rather than the inner edge? Whenever the foot is touching the ground—even with no weight on it—the alignment should be optimal for bearing full weight, which might suddenly become necessary. Applying full or even partial weight to the inner edge of the foot, as in Figure 10-5b, could cause a sprain of the ankle. From a martial standpoint, an empty, non-centered foot is quite vulnerable to attack.

---

7. Robert Chuckrow, *The Tai Chi Book* (Wolfeboro, NH: YMAA Publication Center, 1998), 178.

Practicing Stepping to the Side Using a Movement from the Taiji Form

"Preparation" and the Evolution from Wuji to Taiji

The first movement, "Preparation," of the Cheng Man-ch'ing short form is of paramount importance. It incorporates the basic Taoist philosophy of Taiji, namely, the evolution of Wuji (nothingness) into Taiji (the separation, balance, exchange, and continuous interchange of *yin* and *yang*). In fact, the *yin-yang* exchange embodied in "Preparation" stepping is the prototype for *all* the myriad ways of stepping in the form.

Practicing "Preparation"

The following is how to practice this movement in a manner that is consistent with the Tai-Chi principles.

Stand facing north (where, again, the starting direction is arbitrarily defined to be north) with heels lightly touching, feet angled out comfortably, and arms simply hanging at the sides (Wuji) (Fig. 10-7*a*). Next, lower your body by shifting your weight 100 percent onto your right foot, creating a constraint that as your body sinks, it correspondingly turns to the right. As your left foot empties, its heel automatically lifts slightly, and that foot rotates outward about its ball as a result of the turning of your body (Fig. 10-7*b*).

As you sink into your right leg, it becomes increasingly *yin* (yielding, earthy, downward, inactive, supportive). It is important not to let your body "fall" and be stopped only by the stretching of the quadriceps. Instead, your right leg should have a yang counterpart, which is an upward expansion that continuously regulates the lowering of the body.

As you sink and turn, your arms expand and become slightly bent at the elbows, and your forearms rotate so that both palms face the rear (such rotation is discussed in Experiment 2-4). Also, as you sink, allow a stretched spring in your outwardly-angled right hip joint to release, which turns your body to the right. Your left leg then also turns, pivoting on the ball of your left foot, thereby initiating its outward motion.

As you sink into your right leg, your left leg must become correspondingly *yang*, which means that you are "activating" its bioelectricity to make it increasingly expanded, buoyant, and ready to step westward. That action plus the outward momentum of the turning foot ensures that the moment the weight is 100 percent on the right foot and friction between the foot and the floor becomes zero, the left foot already starts to become airborne.

Of course, the step is not activated from the foot but involves the whole body. Just as "a hand is not a hand," "a foot is not a foot."

All of the weight-bearing parts of the left foot should contact the ground simultaneously, with the weight shifting from zero to 100 percent in a manner similar to that portrayed in Figure 10-2. That is, the left foot must blend with the floor with no discontinuity of movement or pressure.

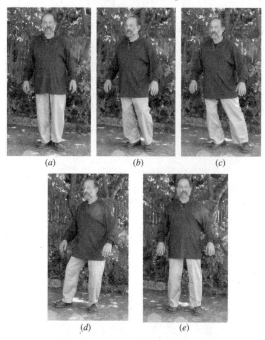

Fig. 10-7. Sequence of "Preparation" of the Cheng Man-ch'ing short form.

In fine-tuning this movement, it is good to view your reflection and that of your surroundings in a mirror. Any sideways movement of your body will be sensitively revealed by a movement of the reflection of your head relative to that of its surroundings. As you step to the side, there should be no movement of your head and body in the direction of the step until after your stepping foot contacts the floor with zero pressure. Only then should the foot blend with the floor. Actually, your body will need to shift slightly in the opposite direction to that of the stepping leg in order to counterbalance its weight and leverage.

Note also that the rotational motion of the left leg evolves into translational motion, thus reducing the effort required.

When the left foot touches the ground, the centerline of that foot should lie on a north-south line (Fig. 10-7c). Next, allow the right thigh joint springs to release, causing your body to shift 100 percent of your weight to the left foot (Fig. 10-7d).

When your body stops shifting, the centerline of your body points northeastward, and your left foot points northward. Thus, the tissues in your left thigh joint are stretched, causing your body to turn counterclockwise about the left hip joint to face the starting direction and also causing the right foot to pivot inward on the heel until its centerline also lies on a north-south line.

As you come to standing 50-50, with feet parallel and knees straight but loose, release as much tension as possible in both hip joints. The palms of the hands face the rear, the elbows are slightly bent, and the thumbs are at the centers of the sides of the thighs. Both feet should be parallel, pointing north, and shoulder width apart. Both heels should lie on an east-west line (Fig. 10-7e).

Comment. It is very important (a) that the left foot start its turning and outward motions as a result of the turning of the body, (b) that you step without any discontinuity in the movement of your left foot, and (c) that the stepping foot blend with the ground continuously and without any premature commitment of weight.

Stepping Naturally

Natural Stepping During Walking

Walking is something that we do on a regular basis, so it is worthwhile to examine how that is naturally done and then extend its elements into Taiji movement. If you watch people walk, you will see that, except for those with a serious impairment, the following manner of leg usage holds: as the body shifts forward, the rearmost leg reaches a point where it would drag on the ground. Just before that point, the knee of that leg is then slightly lifted and naturally swings forward, causing the lower part of that leg and foot to become airborne and swing backward relative to the knee. When the forward motion of the knee stops, the lower leg continues to freely swing forward about the knee as a result of its momentum and pendulum motion of the leg. If the lower leg were not allowed to swing backward, the forward swing would be correspondingly less, and extra energy would be needed to then extend the lower leg for the step.

Unnatural Stepping

An evident error among some Taiji practitioners is that of unnatural movement of their legs during stepping. When stepping, some Taiji practitioners tend to lift and move their legs stiffly, as rigid units, and lead with a foot instead of allowing their upper and lower legs to swing freely, as occurs in everyday walking.

Walking by bringing a whole rear leg forward as a unit requires using excessive energy (which is wasteful and violates the principle of non-action), slows you down, and produces unnecessary vulnerability. The whole leg has much more mass and, when extended, has much more leverage and resistance to a change in movement than does just the upper leg. If allowed to relax, a leg (or an arm) can act as a pendulum. The energy for stepping is then supplied by nature, free of charge.

Other Leg-Movement Possibilities

In much Taiji, not only does the stepping leg move forward, it also arcs out, to the side. Physiologically, walking forward involves only a swiveling action of the hip joints, which is only one of the three independent modes of the movement of that joint. These independent modes involve (1) sagittal, (2) horizontal, and (3) frontal leg movements (see Fig. 10-8, showing the medial, frontal and horizontal planes, noting that a sagittal plane is any plane parallel to the median plane).

Sagittal movement involves a swiveling of the thigh joint and occurs when moving the knee forward and backward, as in walking. Horizontal and frontal movements involve hinge-like opening/closing. Horizontal movement occurs when arcing the knee outward or inward. Frontal movement occurs when you lift a foot inward to look at its sole. Sagittal and horizontal leg movements occur a lot in Taiji. The frontal movement occurs in other martial arts, e.g., the side kick.

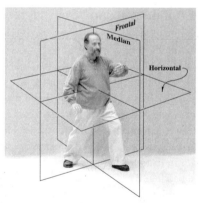

Fig. 10-8. The three planes of the body. A sagittal plane is any plane parallel to the median plane.[8]

A hallmark of Taiji movement is not only the swiveling movement but also the hinge-like opening of the hip joints involved in the horizontal, outward, arcing movement of Taiji stepping. The more extended the leg is while arcing outward, the greater is the amount of strength required for that action for two

8. Figure from Robert Chuckrow, *Tai Chi Dynamics* (Wolfeboro, NH: YMAA Publication Center, 2008), 25–26.

reasons: (1) the more extended, the more leverage, and (2) the more extended, the greater the resistance to angular change in movement. These consequences can be avoided by allowing the lower leg to naturally swing inward while arcing the leg horizontally outward and then allowing the lower leg to naturally swing forward to step.

The Swing of the Rear Leg During Stepping Forward

The stages of the swing of the upper and lower rear leg when it steps forward are shown in Figure 10-9. An example of such movement occurs for the left leg in "Step Forward, Intercept, and Punch."

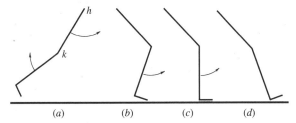

(a) (b) (c) (d)

Fig. 10-9. Stages of the rear leg stepping forward as the hip joint h moves continuously forward during a natural stride (somewhat exaggerated): (a) the rear leg just before stepping forward. As the knee k starts to arc forward, the lower leg lags behind, swinging backward relative to the upper leg; (b) the knee stops, and the lower leg swings forward past (c) to (d); (d) the lower leg has freely swung forward into a position with the heel just touching the ground. No weight has shifted yet. Note that the hip joint h remains stationary throughout the step.

Experiment 10-1. Next time you are in a store where there are chairs or benches in the front, sit down and watch people walk. You may notice people pronating their knees (caving them inward), locking their knees with each step, or angling their feet outward, thereby shifting side to side as they walk. But you will see very few people walking without allowing the natural swing of their legs.

Experiment 10-2. Next time you are in a supermarket or other store, try walking with a shopping cart. The extra stability and possibly support that the cart provides allows you to walk in a much more relaxed manner, allowing the swing of your upper and lower legs to develop naturally. Then capture that feeling and later recreate it as you practice Taiji movement.

Experiment 10-3. Sit on the edge of a sturdy table, with knees just beyond the edge. Lift your lower leg and let it swing. If the muscles in your leg are relaxed, the lower leg will swing forward and back many times with decreasing amplitude, until it finally stops. Then capture the feeling of release and swing, and then experiment with allowing that swing to occur while doing Taiji stepping.

Experiment 10-4. When you walk in daily life, notice how your rear upper leg swings forward before your lower leg swings forward. Then capture that feeling and experiment with that way of stepping while doing Taiji.

The Swing of the Forward Leg During Stepping Forward

Two movements, "Ward Off Left" and "Single Whip," will be discussed in this section. The stages of the swing of the left leg when it steps into "Ward Off Left" and "Single Whip" are shown in Figures 10-10 and 10-11, respectively.

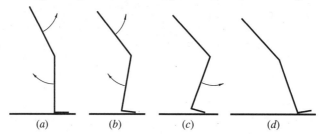

(a)   (b)   (c)   (d)

Fig. 10-10. This example shows four stages of the left leg stepping into "Ward Off Left": (a) the empty leg before taking a step; (b) the weight sinks into the right leg, and the left knee starts to bend; (c) the weight sinks more, and the knee bends more; (d) the knee remains stationary, and the lower leg has freely swung forward into a position with the heel just touching the ground. No weight has shifted yet. Note that the hip joint continually lowers as the rooted leg increasingly bends.

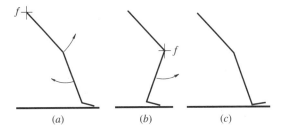

(a)   (b)   (c)

Fig. 10-11. This example shows three stages of the left leg stepping into "Single Whip." Here *f* designates a fixed point. (*a*) the empty left leg before slightly raising the knee and letting the lower leg swing backward about the knee joint; (*b*) the empty left leg after swinging backward about the knee joint and before opening horizontally at the hip joint and then allowing the left lower leg to swing forward about the knee joint; (*c*) the empty left leg after the lower leg swings forward about the knee joint. The heel of the left leg touches the ground after stepping, before shifting the weight.

Stepping at the Right Moment

The key to stepping at the right moment is totally emptying the stepping leg (no commitment of weight) a substantial amount of time before the step occurs. When the stepping foot is totally empty during the transition prior to stepping, at a certain instant, the turning of the body will cause that foot to move, signaling the time for stepping to occur. If there is even the slightest force between the ground and the stepping foot during the transition prior to stepping, friction between that foot and the floor will prevent its movement, and there will be no signal for stepping at the right moment. Moreover, the impetus imparted to the stepping leg to continue its movement will also be lost.

Experiments for Attaining Proper Stepping

Experiment 10-5. Centers of Feet. An important facet of improving balance is an awareness of the centers of the feet. Imagine standing, balanced on one leg, with your foot on a board, supported from below by a pointed, vertical stake. The center of that foot is the point directly above the point of contact of the stake and the board. The center of a foot is always in the same place on the foot and does not depend on the amount of weight on that foot. The goal is to have the center of the weight distribution on each foot located at the center of that foot for any amount of weight on it. Yes, even when there is zero weight on a foot, its alignment should be ready for a transfer of weight onto it without having to make split-second changes.

Experiment 10-6. Stacking of the Three Centers of Mass. Another important facet of balance is vertically lining up the centers of mass of the head, chest, and pelvic region. Then, when standing on one foot, those centers are stacked directly above the center of the weighted foot. When in a 70-30 posture (70 percent of the weight on the forward foot), those centers are stacked over a line joining the centers of the feet, 70 percent of the way from the rear to the front.

Experiment 10-7. Practicing Stepping Forward Using a Movement from the Taiji Form. An excellent exercise for reinforcing the principles of stepping like a cat just outlined is to practice the first movement, "Ward Off Left" (Fig. 10-11), of the Cheng Man-ch'ing short form, described below. In doing this movement, it is important that the left leg swing freely at its knee joint. As you step forward, there should be no movement of your head and body in the direction of the step until after your stepping foot contacts the floor with zero pressure. Only then does the foot blend with the floor.

"Ward Off with Left Hand"

Stand facing north in a 50-50 stance with the palms of the hands facing the rear, the elbows slightly bent, and the thumbs close to the sides of the thighs (Fig. 10-12a). Next, shift the weight 100 percent onto the left foot and sink into that foot. As you sink, create a constraint that results in your body correspondingly turning 45 percent to the right. At the same time the sinking into your left foot contributes to an expansion that raises your right arm, palm-down, along a vertical line. Also, the turning of your body in a unified manner causes your right foot to pivot on its heel to point northeastward. Moreover, the turning of your body to the right causes your left arm to swing slightly to the left, as in Experiments 9-8 and 9-10.

Note that with all the weight on the left foot, the left knee is directly above the centerline of the left foot. Then shift the weight 100 percent onto the right foot. During the time you are shifting, you are actively extending your left knee outward and slightly lifting it by using expansion in the pelvic region. Moreover, the shifting of your body to the right causes your left arm to swing even more so to the left. The tension resulting from the openness of the thigh joints now causes your body to turn slightly to the left. As the weight on the left foot decreases, the left heel automatically rises slightly in preparation for a step. Also, when the weight has finished shifting to the right foot, your left arm naturally swings to your right. The hands end up as if holding a large ball in front of the center of the chest with the right hand above, the left hand below, and both palms facing each other (Fig. 10-12*b*). At the moment that your weight is 100 percent off the left leg (Fig. 10-12*c*), step northward with the left foot by letting the lower leg swing forward, pivoting at the knee (Fig. 10-12*d*).

Next, as the weight shifts 70 percent onto the left foot, the left arm continues its motion, circling upward (Fig. 10-12*e*). At the same time, the right arm lowers back to its starting position with your thumb near your thigh as your body continues turning to face north, simultaneously pivoting the right foot on its heel to point northeastward. At the same time, the left hand continues to circle to a position in front of the center of the chest, palm facing inward, and the right hand moves vertically down, ending up with the palm facing the rear near the right thigh (Fig. 10-12*f*). The arms are "rounded as if propped up" (an admonition emphasized by Yang Cheng-fu).[9]

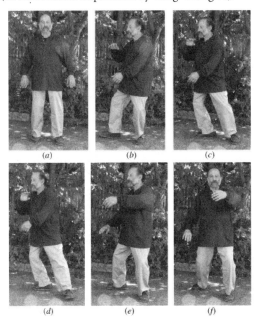

Fig. 10-12. Sequence of "Ward Off Left" of the Cheng Man-ch'ing short form.

In the resources mentioned in the footnotes below, view a video of *yin* and *yang* in "Ward Off"[10] and a video of the energetics of Ward-Off stepping.[11]

---

9. Douglas Wile, comp. and trans., *T'ai Chi Touchstones: Yang Family Secret Transmissions* (Brooklyn, NY: Sweet Ch'i Press, 1983), 65.

10. https://www.chuckrowtaichi.com/YinYangInWardOff.mp4.

11. https://www.chuckrowtaichi.com/AdductorExpansion.mp4.

Comments: One of the most common errors made by beginners is that of losing the width of the stance during stepping. It is essential that the left knee point northward while stepping. If that knee caves inward (points northeastward) instead of pointing in the starting direction, the step will also be inward at the expense of the width of the stance. Note that in going from (*b*) to (*c*) in Figure 10-12, the left leg tilts forward as a unit in its correct alignment.

Swing of the Arms During Walking

It is said that the backward swing of an arm during walking as the leg on that side steps forward is a result of a rotation of the pelvis about a vertical axis. I have come to some conclusions from watching many people at different angles and noting the movements (if any) of different parts of their bodies.

Almost none of the people I have observed rotate their hips any appreciable amount about a vertical axis while walking.

Regarding the opposing motion of the arm and leg on each side, I conclude that the arm swing is active rather than passively resulting from the motion of the pelvis or leg. The purpose of the movement of an arm is to counterbalance the opposite movement of the leg in order to stabilize the body and keep it from turning. I have tried walking with my arms hanging lifelessly, and they do not swing at all or do swing but in a varying fashion relative to the movements of my legs.

The active swing of the arms during running is similar to that during walking, but the arms need to move more vigorously to counterbalance.

Think about it; it would be a waste of energy for the whole body to rotate back and forth while walking when the arms can accomplish the counterbalancing action by using almost no energy.

Chapter 11

Periodic Movement and Its Timing

The subject matter of this chapter is of value in attaining the health, timing, efficiency, naturalness, and martial aspects of Taiji. Feeling the timing that maximizes the successive transfer of motion from your legs to all parts of your body and out to your arms is a precursor to optimally coupling your motion to that of a partner or opponent, whether that be a push or a strike.

Periodic Motion

Periodic (vibratory) motion, which is a regularly repeating, to-and-fro motion, is a common occurrence in nature. Examples are a pendulum or a mass attached to the bottom of a hanging spring. Even bridges are susceptible to vibrations that are large enough to cause them to collapse.[1] For that reason, soldiers never march when crossing bridges.

Two aspects are required for a system to undergo periodic motion: an inertial aspect and an elastic restoring force. For a spring-mass system, the spring supplies the restoring force. For a pendulum, the restoring force is the horizontal component of the tension in the string.

The spring-mass manifests one-dimensional motion (motion along a straight line), and the pendulum manifests two-dimensional motion (motion in a plane). Both of these two periodic motions frequently occur (or should occur) in Taiji movement, as will be discussed later in this chapter.

> **Experiment 11-1.** Repeat Experiment 10-3, feeling the swing of your legs while sitting on the edge of a table.

---

1. Tacoma Narrows Bridge Collapse: https://www.youtube.com/watch%3Fv%3Dj-zcz JXSxnw.

In nature, vibrations can be so slow that the period, which is the time for one complete vibration of to-and-fro movement, is on the order of tens of years. An example of such a slow vibration is the nutation of the earth's axis, which is a to-and-fro wobble of the axis of the yearly rotation of the earth. The nutation of the earth's axis has a period of 18.6 years. In contrast, vibrations can occur quadrillions of times per second. An example of such a high rate of vibration is that of visible light, which has a period on the order of one-qua-drillionth of a second (10^{-15} s). Vibrations whose movement can be followed with our eyes range in frequency from about a few tenths of a second to one hundred seconds.

Periodic Motion Terms

Displacement

Displacement is the distance from equilibrium. Displacements to the right and upward are usually considered to be positive, and displacements to the left and downward are usually considered to be negative.

Amplitude

Amplitude A is the maximum displacement (see Fig. 11-1). A is always positive.

Period

Period T is the time for one complete cycle of a periodic motion. The period in Figure 11-1 is $T = 4$ s.

Frequency

Frequency f is the number of complete cycles per second. The frequency in Figure 11-1 is $f = 1/4$ s.

Note: It can be seen from their definitions that the period and frequency are reciprocally related: $T = 1/f$.

Phase

Phase is the fraction of a complete cycle of a periodic occurrence (can be expressed as a fraction or as an angle). See Figure 11-1 for elucidation of the terms *lead* and *lag*.

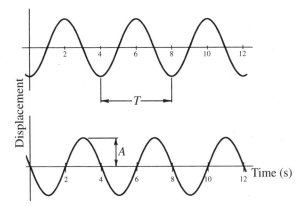

Fig. 11-1. Two displacement-versus-time graphs, each depicting about three cycles of a periodic up-and-down motion of a single particle, of period $T = 4$ seconds (s). The upper motion leads the lower motion by one quarter of a cycle. That is, at time $= 0$, the upper motion has reached its minimum, but the lower motion doesn't reach its minimum until one-quarter of a cycle later (1 s later). Note that the two motions alternate between going with and opposite to each other every successive quarter cycle. Also, when one motion is at its center (zero displacement and maximum motion), the other motion is at its extreme displacement and momentarily stops and changes direction.

To actually see that the upper graph depicts a motion that is ahead of that of the lower one, take a 4" X 6" index card and cut a 1/16-inch-wide, 4-inch-long slot along the middle of the long dimension of the card. Then place the slot vertically over the beginning of the graphs and move the card uniformly to the right. You will then see an up-and-down motion for each through the slot, and the top motion will be seen to lead, with its motion a quarter of a cycle ahead of the lower motion.

Driven Periodic Motion

Natural Frequency

The natural frequency of a system is the rate at which it vibrates or swings to and fro without the influence of an external driving force.

Driven Vibration

When a system is driven by an external vibrational force, it will oscillate at the frequency of the driving force, which may or may not be the natural frequency of the system.

Starting any motion takes force. But once motion is underway, friction dissipates energy. So to maintain a periodic motion of steady amplitude, or to increase its amplitude, a driving force is required. There is a maximum transfer of motion to the system when the driving force is at the natural rate of the system, and the motion of the driving force leads that of the system by one-quarter of a cycle. Such a relationship is displayed in Figure 11-1, assuming that the upper motion, which leads the lower motion by one-quarter of a cycle, is that of the driving force.

Experiment 11-2. Hold a pitcher that is half-full of water over a sink and try swirling the water circularly. Note that in this case, the water in the pitcher circles at a rate based on the rate you swirl it and the friction of the water with the container. The water has inertia, but there is no elastic restoring force. Therefore, there is only circular motion and no natural frequency.

Experiment 11-3. Hold an end of a yardstick or other similar length of wood, and let it hang lightly between your thumb and forefinger. With your other hand, displace and then release its lower end and let it swing. Observe its natural frequency. The period should be about one second.

Next, move your hand back and forth to vibrate it at a rate much higher than its natural frequency. Notice that the amplitude will be rather small, and the lower end of the stick will vibrate oppositely to the motion of your hand. Next, try to vibrate it at a rate much lower than its natural frequency.

Notice that the amplitude will be rather small, and the stick will move with your hand and barely vibrate.

Finally, try to vibrate it at its natural frequency, and see how large the amplitude easily becomes.

Observe: (1) When the natural frequency is reached, the amplitude will be greatest when the movement of your hand leads that of the weight by one-quarter of a cycle. (2) When your hand leads by one-quarter of a cycle, you barely need to move it in order to transfer movement to the weight.

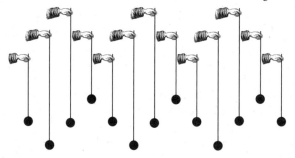

Fig. 11-2. Thirteen successive "snapshots" of a hand holding a rubber band with a weight attached to its lower end and moving periodically up and down at its natural frequency. Shown are three full cycles of up-and-down motion of the hand, which provides the driving force. The snapshots are one-quarter-cycle apart. Note that the motion of the mass lags that of the hand by one-quarter cycle.

Experiment 11-4. Fasten an approximately two-foot-long rubber band or a series of them to a weight such as a fishing sinker (ten ounces works well). Hold the free end of the rubber band between your thumb and forefinger (Fig. 11-2). Then pull the weight down, slightly stretching the rubber band, and release the weight. Observe the natural frequency. Next, try to vibrate it at a rate much higher than its natural frequency. Notice that the vibrational amplitude will be rather small, and the weight will vibrate oppositely to your hand. Next, try to vibrate it at a rate much lower than its natural frequency. Notice that the vibrational amplitude will be rather small, and the weight will move with your hand and barely swing. Finally, try to vibrate it at its natural frequency.

Observe: (1) When the natural frequency is reached, the amplitude will be greatest when the movement of your hand leads that of the weight by one-quarter of a cycle. (2) When your hand leads by one-quarter of a cycle, you barely need to move your hand in order to transfer the movement to the weight.

Linear, Driven, Horizontal Periodic Motion ("Withdraw and Push")

Most Taiji practitioners are familiar with and optimally experience linear, driven, horizontal, periodic motion of the arms in the transition of "Withdraw and Push." In that movement, the arms are supported with the minimum force to neutralize the effect of gravity. The body moves backward, then the arms and hands follow, lagging behind (Fig. 11-3 *a–c*). The body next starts moving forward as the arms are still moving backward relative to the body (Fig. 11-3 *c–e*). Then the body moves backward, with the arms moving forward relative to the body (Fig. 11-3 *e–g*). This relative movement of the body and the arms and hands involves the same timing as that of the vertical movement in Figure 11-3. In "Withdraw and Push," the body provides the driving force, and the restoring force is supplied by the elasticity of the arm, shoulder, and chest tissues in different amounts and at different stages of the motion. In the case of the rubber band and weight, it might seem that gravity is a factor. However, the initial stretch of the rubber band neutralizes gravity, so the motion is analogous to that of "Withdraw and Push."

Analysis of the Motion in "Withdraw and Push"

In Figure 11-3 (*a*) and (*b*), the body moves backward, starting the motion of the arms backward. In Figure 11-3 (*c*), the body has stopped its rearward motion, but the arms are still moving rearward due to their momentum. In

Figure 11-3 (*d*), the body is now moving forward, and the hands are still moving rearward, which starts to compress a spring (the elasticity of the bodily tissues), thereby initiating a forward motion of the arms. From Figure 11-3 (*d*) to (*e*), the arms and body are moving together due to the forward momentum of the arms. In Figure 11-3 (*e*), the body stops, but the arms continue moving forward due to their momentum. At the same time, the body is moving backward, starting to pull the arms rearward.

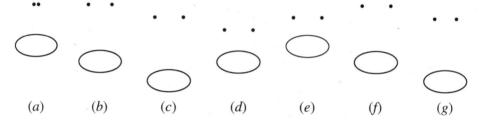

(*a*)　　(*b*)　　(*c*)　　(*d*)　　(*e*)　　(*f*)　　(*g*)

Fig. 11-3. Successive "snapshots," as viewed from above, of the body and hands in the transition from "Press" to "Withdraw and Push." Each oval and pair of dots above it represent the body and hands, respectively. The snapshots *a–g* are one-quarter cycle apart. Note that after the motion starts, the motion of the hands lags that of the body by one-quarter cycle.

Experiment 11-5. Do the movement "Withdraw and Push" repeatedly, feeling the natural rate of the forward and backward movement of the arms when supported by only the minimum strength to keep them from falling. Do not allow tension or a preconceived idea of the movement to interfere. The shoulders and elbows must be as relaxed as possible.

Observe: (1) When the natural frequency is reached, the amplitude will be greatest when the movement of your body leads that of the hands by one-quarter of a cycle. (2) When your body leads that of the hands by one-quarter of a cycle, the transfer of movement to the arms is greatest. For that relationship, your body starts moving forward when your hands are halfway to the rear, and your body starts moving backward when your hands have moved halfway forward.

Importance of Timing of "Withdraw and Push"

Feeling the optimal timing of the propulsion of your own bodily parts is necessary in order to naturally achieve a corresponding timing in pushing a partner in push-hands practice or in responding to an opponent's attack. If you can't feel that timing in your own body, how are you going to produce the effect in coupling your movement with that of another person?

Circular Motion of Right Arm in "Single Whip"

"Single Whip" is one of the most fascinating and complex movements in the empty-hand Taiji form. Perhaps that is why it occurs so frequently—eleven times in the Yang long form.[2]

The transition of "Single Whip" before stepping with the left foot involves a simultaneous circular movement of the right hand in the horizontal plane and one of the left hand in the frontal plane. An important feature of this transition is the timing of the turning of the trunk of the body relative to that of the arms to maximize the transfer of movement from the feet, to the body, to the arms (see Fig. 11-4 for the optimal timing for the right arm).

Interestingly, the optimal timing of the turning of the trunk of the body to maximize the movement of the right arm is exactly the same as that for the left arm. Moreover, that timing is exactly the same for all motions of arms in all parts of the form, whether the movement is frontal, sagittal, or horizontal. The universality of that relationship suggests that all of the movements of the form were expected to occur with that consideration in mind.

Once you have learned to time the turning of the body relative to that of the arm(s) for circular motion in the horizontal plane (as in the case of the right hand in the transition into "Single Whip"), then apply that timing to circular motion in the frontal and sagittal planes (see Fig. 10-8, which illustrates the three planes).

---

2. For occurrences and comparisons of movements in both the Yang and Cheng Man-ch'ing forms, visit https://www.chuckrowtaichi.com/CMCvsYang.html.

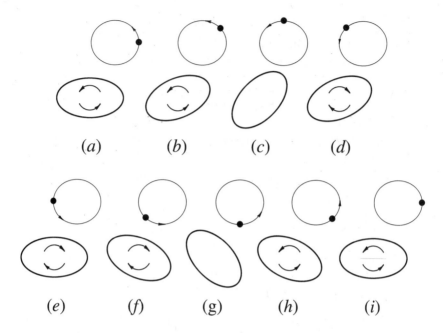

(a) (b) (c) (d)

(e) (f) (g) (h) (i)

Fig. 11-4. Successive "snapshots," as viewed from above, of the horizontal motion of the right hand during the transition into "Single Whip" before stepping with the left foot. The snapshots are one-quarter cycle apart. Note that the motion of the body (an oval) leads that of the hand (a dot) by one-quarter of a cycle. Note that the direction of rotation of the body changes when the hand is midway between one side and the other of its circular motion.

Experiment 11-6 (frontal movement). Do the movement "Cloud Hands" repeatedly in a 50-50 stance without stepping. Feel the natural rate of turning of the body to maximize the frontal movement of the arms. Shoulders and elbows must be as relaxed as possible.

Experiment 11-7 (sagittal movement). Do the movement "Roll Back and Press" repeatedly, feeling the natural rate of turning of the body to maximize the sagittal movement of the arm. Shoulders and elbows must be as relaxed as possible.

Experiment 11-8 (horizontal movement). Do the movement "Single Whip" repeatedly, feeling the natural rate of turning of the body to maximize the horizontal movement of the right arm. Shoulders and elbows must be as relaxed as possible.

Centrifugal Effect

An object undergoing circular motion experiences an acceleration toward its center, called *centripetal acceleration*. Whenever there is an acceleration, there must be a force, called *centripetal force*, in the direction of the acceleration. Thus, in order for an object to move in a circle, there must be a force on it toward the center. If the centripetal force is removed, the object will move off along a line that is tangential to the circle. Viewed from a frame of reference rotating at the same rate as the object, the object will seem to act as though there were a force on it away from the center (called *centrifugal force*).

When you are a passenger in a car rounding a curve, you feel as though there is a force away from the center of rotation. The seat belt and possibly the door supply the centripetal force to keep you in place.

Similarly, when you rotate your body with your arms hanging, unless you hold your arms inward, they will tend to move outward and, therefore, rise. This effect can be experienced in some movements of the form such as "Single Whip" when done sufficiently quickly.

> **Experiment 11-9.** With your arms hanging and totally relaxed, alternately rotate your body right and left about a fixed, vertical axis through the center of the body. As you increase the rate of back-and-forth turning, notice that your arms tend to increasingly separate from your body and rise as they rotate circularly.

Centrifugal Effect with Gravity

Professor Cheng had us do "Roll Back and Press" by circling the left arm fully downward in a sagittal circle. Others do that movement in an almost horizontal plane. Professor Cheng's way promotes increased relaxation at the bottom of the circle. But there is another benefit, intended or not. Namely, when any mass rotates in a vertical circle, the centrifugal and gravitational effects add at the bottom. The centrifugal effect is always radially away from the center, which at the bottom is downward and in the same direction as the force of gravity. The addition of both those effects at the bottom of the circle thus produce a noticeably large hydraulic pressure in the hand and forearm. One result beyond relaxation is an increase in the "washing" effect discussed in Chapter 9.

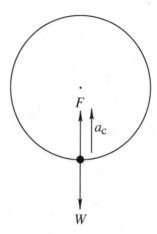

Fig. 11-5. Forces on a typical droplet of water in the hand at the lowest point of its circular motion in a vertical plane.

Figure 11-5 depicts the forces on a typical droplet of water in the hand at the lowest point of its circular motion in a vertical plane. W is the gravitational force acting on the droplet, and a_c is the acceleration of the droplet toward the center of the circular motion. We can write the equation of motion as follows:

$$\Sigma F = ma_c$$
$$F - W = ma_c$$
$$F = W + ma_c$$

Thus, the upward force on the droplet at the bottom is greater than its weight by an amount ma_c. This upward force is provided by the tissues, which therefore experience a greater than normal pressure. In addition, if the tissues are relaxed and "liquefied," there is a hydraulic pressure gradient in the whole arm, which is greatest when the arm is hanging. These three factors (weight, centrifugal effect, and hydraulic pressure) add to increase the swelling and pressurizing of the tissues of the hand.

Conical Pendulum

A simple pendulum, consisting of a string attached to a weight, which swings to and fro in a vertical plane, can instead be used as a conical pendulum, whose bob rotates circularly in a horizontal plane (Fig. 11-6). The *conical pendulum* is so named because the string describes a cone.

In this case, the horizontal component of the tension in the string supplies the force toward the center that keeps the mass moving circularly rather than tangentially off the circular path. The vertical component of tension in the string balances the weight of the mass.

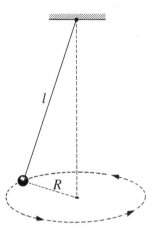

Fig. 11-6. A conical pendulum.

> **Experiment 11-10.** Try moving your body so that your shoulder moves circularly in a horizontal plane about a fixed vertical axis, with one arm hanging and circling at its natural rate (conical pendulum). Notice that your body leads the motion of the arm by one-quarter of a cycle. It is essential to relax your arm and shoulder in order to experience the natural motion.

"Swinging"—Turning the Body about a Vertical Axis, Arms Swinging Side to Side

This exercise is a precursor to *fajin* (a whip-like, explosive energy release). It is different from the "Constant Bear," taught by Prof Cheng, which involves shifting side to side and turning, thereby causing the arms to swing.

This swinging exercise involves standing in either a 50-50, feet-parallel stance, or a 50-50 bow stance (not 70-30). The arms move totally passively, resulting only from the alternating turning of the body to one side and to the other about a stationary vertical axis.

The head always points in the neutral direction, floating as the body turns underneath. As the body turns from one side to the other, the centrifugal effect causes the arms to rise to an almost horizontal motion, and they swing side-to-side and hit the front, sides, and back of the body as a result of the turning.

An important goal of swinging is to maximize the transfer of motion of the turning of the body to the arms. Non-action (minimum effort, maximum effect) occurs when the arms move the most for the smallest motion of the hips. Two elements are necessary: (1) turning the body at the natural rate of the swing of the arms and (2) timing the turning of the body to *lead* (move earlier than) the swinging of the arms by a quarter of a cycle (see Figure 11-7*a–i* for the evolution corresponding to a whole cycle). This quarter-cycle phase relationship between the "driving force" and the motion is well known in physics and is a standard topic in an intermediate physics course.

To get a feeling for the timing of the turning of the body relative to the motion of the arms, visualize a dog shaking off water. In the footnoted slow-motion video below,[3] the motion of the dog's jowls and ears are analogous to that of your arms in side-to-side swinging. Note how the direction of rotation of the dog's head reverses when an ear is pointed straight upward (at the middle of its back-and-forth motion). The puppies don't seem to have it down yet.

Benefits of Swinging

As you become proficient in achieving the optimal timing of the turning of the trunk of your body to the movement of your arms, the intensity of arm movement dramatically increases for the energy and movement required. Maximizing such efficiency produces the following benefits.

Health

The arms hitting the body with considerable intensity, called *therapeutic tapping*, increases circulation of *qi*, blood, and lymph, with their associated nutritive, cleansing, and healing qualities. The beneficial vibration produced extends to the organs, glands, bones, blood vessels, and nerves in the trunk of the body and arms. Also the jostling and passive movement of the shoulder and chest muscles conduce to an increase in *qi* in those regions.

Reduction in Need for Contractive Strength

Habituation to the use of contractive strength is a barrier to recognition of expansive strength. In doing the movements of the form, maximizing the transfer of mechanical energy to the arms from the optimal timing of the turning of the body reduces the need for muscular strength to lift the arms against gravity. Thus, learning the use of expansive strength is accelerated.

---

3. https://www.youtube.com/watch?v=HVe5caFCUrE.

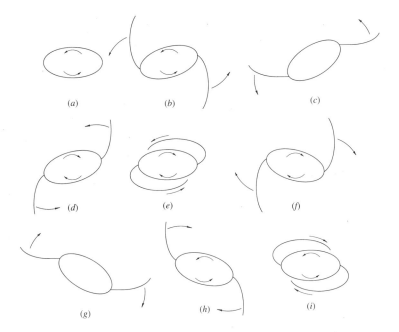

Fig. 11-7. Top view of one full cycle of swinging about a vertical axis. At optimal transfer of turning motion of the body (oval) to the arms (curved lines), the arms *lag* (move later than) the body by one-quarter cycle. (*a*) Body in neutral state and starting to turn counterclockwise, arms hanging and lagging because of their inertia. (*b*) Body turned 15 degrees counterclockwise from neutral, continuing to turn counterclockwise, with arms having stopped lagging and now starting to move counterclockwise, following the movement of body, and upward as a result of the centrifugal effect. (*c*) Body turned 30 degrees counterclockwise and momentarily not moving, with arms catching up with body and continuing to move counterclockwise of their momentum. (*d*) Body turned 15 degrees counterclockwise, having changed direction of turning to clockwise, with arms continuing to move counterclockwise of their momentum. (*e*) Body facing neutral direction and turning clockwise, arms moving counterclockwise, hitting body. (*f*) Body turned 15 degrees clockwise, continuing to turn clockwise, with arms now moving clockwise, lagging behind movement of body. (*g*) Body turned 30 degrees clockwise and momentarily not moving, with arms catching up with body and continuing to move clockwise of their momentum. (*h*) Body turned 15 degrees clockwise, having changed direction of turning to counterclockwise, with arms continuing to move clockwise. (*i*) Body facing neutral direction and turning counterclockwise, arms moving clockwise, hitting body.

Once you become proficient in attaining the proper timing in horizontal movement, which is easiest, then you should strive to apply it to sagittal and frontal movement (see Fig. 10-8).

Training "Taking Punches"

One of the methods for training the ability of a particular region of the body to be hit without injury involves repetitively tapping that region. I was exposed to such training under William C. C. Ch'en in the late 1970s. Ch'en is famous for his imperviousness and would periodically invite his students and outside martial artists to hit him with full power. Lou Kleinsmith, a senior student of Professor Cheng in New York, said that punching Ch'en is "like hitting a truck tire." My limiting factor was how hard I could hit him without injuring myself. When hit, Ch'en never shows any sign of having been harmed.

Wang Shu-chin (1904–1981) was famous for taking punches and can be seen doing so in this video.[4] The first of the two men punching Wang appears to be Robert Smith (1926–2011).[5] It is said that Wang invited Joe Louis to punch him with full power, but Louis declined, saying that he didn't want to kill Wang by accident.[6]

If you lightly tap the "trained" region of a person who is adept in taking punches, you can feel the tissues instantly "jump" into action against your tap. Such a response is usually absent in an untrained person.

The underlying mechanism of the conditioning seems to be that, when tapped repeatedly, the bodily tissues "learn" to involuntarily expand and solidify when hit. Such expansion and solidification might possibly be produced by bio piezoelectricity.[7] Piezoelectricity is electricity produced by certain materials when subjected to pressure, and it has been found that structural elements of the human body composed of proteins, nucleic acids, and mucopolysaccharides are capable of transducing mechanical energy into an electric current.[8]

With repetitive training, this piezoelectric reaction to tapping might become increasingly efficient at electrically changing water within and surrounding bodily tissues into a gel (see Chapter 2), thereby protecting the body against powerful strikes.

Developing Fajin

In a self-defense modality, small unified excursions send a wave through the body, causing the arms to have large, relaxed, explosive movement, ending in a strike involving the power of the whole body, connected as a unit. The

---

4. https://www.youtube.com/watch?v=TgSPsiQhAZk.
5. https://en.wikipedia.org/wiki/Robert_W._Smith_(writer).
6. https://en.wikipedia.org/wiki/Wang_Shujin.
7. The prefix *piezo* comes from the Greek *piezein*, meaning *to press*.
8. https://www.ncbi.nlm.nih.gov/pubmed/577004.

application of force initiated internally is much less likely to be observed by an opponent than that initiated externally. Internal force originates in the feet, then the legs, and then the turning of the hips, sending a wave through the body. Such movement is responsible in large part for the highly successful, deceptive aspect of Taijiquan as an internal martial art (strength concealed in softness).

Fajin, or energy release, is used for striking in a self-defense modality and is especially emphasized in Chen-style Taijiquan. Chen Taijiquan is the original style, which alternates soft with explosive *fajin* movement. Most practitioners of the Yang style are not taught *fajin*. The likely reason for this omission is that after Yang Lu-chan (1799–1872),[9] the founder of the Yang system, learned Taijiquan from the Chen family, he was summoned by the imperial court to teach Taiji to the imperial family and their bodyguards. To do so, he needed to remove some of the secret elements and make it more suitable for that setting. Once Taiji became public, his goal and that of his successors has been to maximize the spread of Taiji. Such popularization also involves limiting the teaching of elements that would be especially difficult to learn and, thereby, reduce its popularity.

Ti Fang

Ti fang is an action whereby an opponent is caused to lose his root and is then sent flying with the use of minimal force. In order to be effective, *ti fang* requires precise timing of the neutralization and direction of the push. It should be noted that Cheng Man-ch'ing named the Taiji school on 87 Bowery, New York City, Shí Zhòng, which implies appropriate timing, distancing, and direction (Fig. 11-8).

Ti fang begins after the opponent (or partner in push-hands practice) exerts force on you or you exert force on him or her. In either case, you neutralize the force, which means reducing it through judicious movement. The resulting reduction in pressure causes the opponent to slightly lose his balance and move forward. In order to regain his balance, the opponent then presses the ground with the ball and toes of his forward foot, thereby rotating his body slightly backward.

The appropriate timing for your push is at the moment your partner puts weight on his forward foot to pull back from falling forward. The goal is to feel that moment and add your push to your partner's backward movement. If the push is too late, your partner will have already regained balance and root. If the push is too early, your partner will not have sufficiently lost balance and will be rooted.

---

9. https://en.wikipedia.org/wiki/Yang_Luchan.

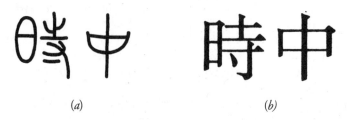

(a)   *(b)*

Fig. 11-8. The characters (*a*) ancient, (*b*) recent, for Shí Zhòng, which were used by Professor Cheng Man-ch'ing in naming his Taiji school. The first character, shí, has a symbol θ on the left representing the sun. In ancient times, the Chinese used a sun dial to know the time. The symbol just to the right of the sun represents a Buddhist temple, whose bells announced the hour. The symbol for the Buddhist temple has a plant 坐 sprouting from the earth and a hand ⇒\ below it, with a horizontal line pointing to the pulse point. The plant suggests upward growth over time, and the pulse also suggests time. The line pointing to the pulse point, which is one inch below the wrist, suggests proper placement. The second character, zhòng, represents a bow and arrow 中, suggesting the idea of aiming in the right direction. Thus, the name, Shí Zhòng, represents the cultivation of appropriate timing, placement, and direction, which are essential elements in Taiji.[10]

---

10. This interpretation of Shi Zhong was explained to me by Ed Young.

Chapter 12

Additional Physical Concepts

Constraints

As used here, a *constraint* is a condition or set of conditions that predetermine a specific intermotion of a physical system. For example, a bead sliding on a straight wire is constrained to move only in a straight line (along the wire) and can also rotate about the wire. Another example is a ceiling-fan blade, which is constrained to rotate about a fixed vertical axis with no other movement. Figure 12-1 shows a "Yankee" screwdriver whose blade is constrained to rotate when the handle is depressed. One more example is a wheel rolling without slipping down an inclined track. The constraint here is that the center of the wheel moves along a line parallel to the incline, and as we will later show, each time the wheel rotates once, it translates a distance equal to its circumference (Fig. 12-2). Other examples of constraints abound.

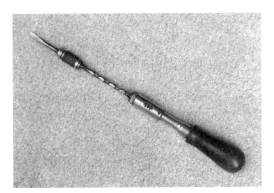

Fig. 12-1. A "Yankee" screwdriver. The chuck holding the screwdriver blade is constrained to rotate clockwise as the handle is pressed inward with one hand while the other hand holds the knurled, freely rotating sleeve next to the chuck. The helical grooves on the shaft are crisscrossed so that sliding the tab on the steel body toward the handle constrains the bit to turn counterclockwise, thereby loosening a screw. The middle position of the tab prevents internal rotation.

Also, by constraining a line in the body to be unchanging except for its rotation about a fulcrum, we can create a lever in any direction in three-dimensional space that can be used in rooting, as described in Experiment 8-1.

Here is an example of a constraint in human interaction: I was at my dentist. He was holding a mirror between my cheek and a molar. Without even slightly changing the position of the mirror, he turned his body and reached for a tool with his other hand. If he hadn't constrained his hand that was holding the mirror to remain in exactly the same position, the mirror could have injuriously pushed against the soft tissue in my mouth.

Constraints in Taiji Movement

It is useful to apply the idea of a constraint to certain motions in Taiji. In such movement, a major goal is to use the least strength possible so that the movements arise maximally from natural effects, namely, alignment, gravity, momentum, angular momentum, inertia, centrifugal effect, and the compression and stretching of bodily springs (elasticity of bodily tissues). However, without the idea (*yi*) of the movement, not much would occur that resembles Taiji movement.

Because the principle of non-action is so essential to Taiji, it is important that we utilize constraints to achieve natural effects rather than contriving the movement to occur from a preconceived idea of timing and position by using contractive force. Such a preconception arises from the *yi* (the idea of the movement) superseding its role. Instead, there should be an appropriate combination of the *yi*, the principles, and awareness of the natural bodily feeling.

It is important to know just how much you are causing an action to occur, the manner in which you are doing so, and the extent to which natural forces are involved. Otherwise, how will you know how to move naturally and with maximum efficiency?

An Example of a Constraint in the Taiji Form

In "Ward Off Left," as the right hand rises and then lowers, you can imagine the wrist to be sliding upward in a vertical slot or on a vertical wire through the wrist joint as a result of the turning of the body. Then the right wrist moves downward along that same slot or wire. In a similar manner, the left arm arcs upward and outward within a circular "slot" as a result of a combination of the shifting and turning of the body and of expansive strength.

Whereas using the image of a slot or wire has value, it should be recognized that that value is limited and short-lived (see "Dangers of Overusing Images in Movement Arts" in Chapter 15).

Constraints in Self-Defense

The relationship of constraints and natural movement to self-defense is quite important. When an opponent attempts to contact your body, it is essential that he not perceive that you are attempting to thwart him. As soon as you oppose the opponent's movement, say by blocking or pulling away, he will become alerted, escalate his strength, and change what he is doing. That change renders valueless much of the prior information you have gained about his attack because everything is now changed.

Instead, if you let the opponent feel that he is succeeding in attaining exactly what he wants, he will become overconfident and possibly be in the future by thinking, "I've got him." Then he will become overextended and, therefore, vulnerable. So your response to his attack must evolve in a subtle way based on a judicious array of constraints that guide his attack safely (deflection of four ounces) as you move appropriately off the line of the attack.

> **Experiment 12-1.** Opponent steps forward and tries to grab your neck. Without loss of generality, assume that he uses his right hand. As his hand approaches, intercept his wrist with the outside of your right wrist so it touches and follows his as you step back with and shift onto your left foot, thereby shifting back and to your left. The constraint here is that even though your body moves to the left, your hand nevertheless leads his hand straight back so it misses your neck. The timing of your movement is crucial. If you move back too early, the opponent will change. If you move to late, he will get your neck.

In a real situation, the proper time to move is not when the opponent has the thought, "I'm going to get him," but when that thought *prematurely* changes to, "I've got him." At that latter point, the opponent is in the future, which means the present goes by, and the opponent is then in the past and vulnerable

> **Experiment 12-2.** Opponent steps forward and grabs your right wrist. Without loss of generality, assume that he uses his right hand. Try each of the following two scenarios:
>
> **1. Worst-case scenario: you don't move as he grabs.** Before doing anything else, gently cover his hand with the palm of your left hand. Doing so prevents his unexpectedly releasing your wrist and striking with that hand. Next, step back diagonally with your right foot, turning to the right as you do so. This action leads the opponent into his weakness, namely, along the line perpendicular to the line joining the centers of his feet. At the same time, your left hand stays with his right hand (constraint) even as your body shifts and turns, and your right hand rotates outward, thereby opening the gate, which is the space between his thumb and forefinger. Now you are free.
>
> *(continued on next page)*

2. Higher-level scenario: you move as he grabs. Now that you can deal with the worst-case scenario, moving as you are grabbed makes your escape much easier. As the opponent reaches for your wrist, you are already stepping and moving back, drawing him into his weakness. Now as you use the prior method, everything is the same except that his grip on your wrist will be weaker or absent. It is essential that the connection between your wrist and his hand is not broken even when no physical contact has yet been made.

Rolling Without Slipping

When a wheel rolls without slipping, it rotates once about its center each time its center translates a length equal to the circumference of the wheel. To see this relationship, imagine a roll of thin double-sided adhesive tape rolling on a flat surface (Fig. 12-2). When a length of tape equal to the circumference of the roll is laid down, the roll of tape must have undergone one complete rotation.

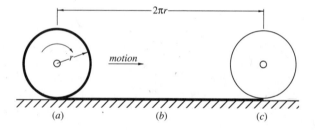

Fig. 12-2. A wheel of radius *r*, rolling without slipping translates its circumference for every complete rotation: (*a*) wheel with one turn of tape (thickness exaggerated); (*b*) length of tape rolled off, laid down, and sticking to the ground; and (*c*) wheel after one 360-degree turn of tape is completely removed. Distance between centers is one circumference ($2\pi r$).

In many of the movements of the Taiji empty-hand form, the final turning motion of the body is accompanied by a simultaneous rotation of one or more wrists (e.g., "Single Whip," "White Crane," "Withdraw and Push," and "Four Corners"). This action is consistent with the Qigong energetics and self-defense applications.

Regarding Qigong, when the rotations away from equilibrium and back are done by releasing contractive strength and expanding and condensing, the acupuncture meridians are beneficially activated.

Regarding self-defense, instead of blocking the opponent, which causes him to stop and reformulate a fresh attack, he is "rolled" along the line of his attack *as you move safely off that line.* By your rolling the opponent, he unexpectedly moves farther than he might have initially intended, thereby causing him to overextend and become vulnerable. The rolling motion can also be utilized to bring you closer to the attacker's body.

The following elements are required for maximizing the effectiveness of such a rolling defense: (1) minimizing the force you exert on the opponent so he feels that he is accomplishing his goal (thwarting his movement alerts him that he is being led), (2) stepping or shifting off the line of the attack at the right time and in the right amount, (3) appropriately regulating the rotations of your arms and body in their timing and relative amounts, and (4) minimizing the movement of your body and arms (knowing when the attack has been neutralized and not going beyond). These elements will be further treated in Chapters 13 and 14.

Rolling Without Slipping in Push-Hands and Form Movements

In push-hands practice, neutralization of your partner's push requires shifting and turning. Your partner should feel that his or her push has moved you instead of your having initiated the movement. That feeling is one of pushing a spherical object that easily translates and turns, based on how it is pushed (like a log floating in the water). Your job is to relax your hip, ankle, and knee joints as much as possible so your body moves freely. Of course, that is the *yin* aspect of the movement. The dot of *yang* in the *yin* just described is to feel how much your turning actively leads your partner off your center and beyond without his or her awareness.

Instead, if you initiate turning or other movement using your eyes and analytical mind, a skilled partner will be immediately alerted and provided with information for locating your center and the inner tension that initiated that movement. Such knowledge can then be used to uproot you.

Experiment 12-3. You will need a cooperative push-hands partner for this experiment.

As your partner pushes you (purposely slightly off your center), arrange everything in your body so that the push turns you at exactly the rate that would happen if you were inanimate. It should not feel to your partner that you are trying to do something. Then alternately reverse roles.

Next, as your partner pushes you (again purposely slightly off center), intentionally move your body, actively rotating the push off. Your partner should now sense that you are using your analytical mind to evade being pushed. Then alternately exchange roles.

> **Experiment 12-4.** Repeat Experiment 12-3, this time finding the smallest amount of shifting and turning that will gently neutralize your partner's push. There should be a verbal dialog with your partner to confirm that the neutralization was both successful and minimal.

There is an expression, "The wrist is the second waist." That is, in many of the movements of the form and those of push-hands, the turning of the wrist corresponds to and augments that of the waist. This action is similar to that of the "ladder of rollers" used to transfer cartons of goods from a delivery truck to the loading dock of a supermarket. When the rotation of the wrist matches the movement of an oncoming push, much less turning of the body is needed to roll off your opponent or partner in push-hands. Again, one full rotation of the wrist is one wrist's circumference more movement that can be used in neutralization.[1]

> **Experiment 12-5.** Involve a cooperative push-hands partner and an additional observer, if available.
>
> Start with the palm of your outstretched hand facing you and your partner contacting the back of your wrist with the palm of his hand. As your partner pushes you, just turn without rotating your wrist, and observe or have an additional person observe how much your partner's hand has moved. Actually, without your rotating your wrist, it will automatically rotate the same number of degrees as that of your body.
>
> Next repeat, rotating your body as before but this time actively rotating your wrist, thumb downward, so its rotation now adds to that of your body. Then observe or have an additional person observe how much more your partner's hand and body have moved.

> **Experiment 12-6.** Do some movements of the form, noting the rotation of the wrists as you move. Movements such as "Ward Off," "Crane Spreads Wings," "Carry Tiger to Mountain," and "Four Corners" especially have wrist rolling movements consistent with their self-defense applications. In fact, the direction of such rolling helps to reveal the application of each movement. Depending on its direction, the rotation of the wrists assists the motion of the opponent away from you or your movement into the opponent's space.

---

1. See video of Chen Shih-hsing (Chen Shixing) emphasizing rotating wrist with the turning of the body in demonstrating Taiji applications (4:19–5:50): https://www.youtube.com/watch?v=uA-4gPb3tfo.

Chapter 13

A Clarification of "Secret" Teachings Revealed by Cheng Man-ch'ing[1]

For quite a few years, I read and reread Professor Cheng's *Cheng Tzu's Thirteen Treatises*.[2] I consider most of this book to contain valuable information. However, even though my Ph.D. is in physics, I found Treatise 7, entitled "Strength and Physics," very hard to understand. Treatise 7 ends with Professor Cheng saying,

> This treatise reveals the secret of many generations of Taijiquan masters. I hope the practitioner will pay special attention to this!

Professor Cheng evidently considered this essay, which deals with neutralization, to be very important and chose to use physics as the main expository tool.

Interestingly, there is a similar section on the physics of Taiji in a book by Yearning K. Chen (1906–1980).[3] Because I was unable to understand that section, I decided that the only way for me to grasp the important subject matter of both writers was to recast it in my own words. That endeavor, which follows, was very fruitful and greatly expanded my understanding of neutralization.

---

1. The material of this chapter was originally published as an article: Robert Chuckrow, "A Clarification of 'Secret' Teachings Revealed by Cheng Man-ch'ing," *Qi: The Journal of Traditional Eastern Health & Fitness* 20, no. 4 (Winter, 2010).
2. Cheng Man-ch'ing, *Cheng Tzu's Thirteen Treatises on T'ai Chi Ch'uan*, trans. Benjamin Pang Jen Lo and Martin Inn (Berkeley, CA: North Atlantic Books, 1981), Ch. 7.
3. Yearning K. Chen, *Tai-Chi Chuan: Its Effects and Practical Applications* (Van Nuys, CA: New Castle Publishing Co., 1979), 15–17.

Basic Concepts

Roundness and Expansiveness

Every point of the outer surface of the body (trunk and limbs) must have an expansive, round quality and feel to the opponent like the surface of an impenetrable sphere. The nature of a sphere is such that its surface at each point is perpendicular to the radius to that point. A skilled opponent will automatically try to make contact with a part of your body on a line straight to your center. It is essential that you shift and turn so that contact is made at an angle to the spherical surface. However, when any part of your body exerts force on an opponent, the direction of that force should always be radially outward from the center of your body. The reason for these conditions will be explained later in this chapter.

Triangles

To make the body into a sphere is an impossible task. However, it is important to realize that the opponent has contacted us only at certain points. It is thus sufficient to simulate a spherical shape only at the points of contact. As mentioned, any force you exert at a point of contact must be outward from your center to that point, and the surface of your body at each point of contact must be perpendicular to the line joining your center and that point (see Fig. 13-1). For two points of contact, there will be two lines, each joining your center with a point of contact. For three points, there will be three lines, and so on. If a line is drawn joining any two points of contact, a triangle is formed with its apex at the body's center. As the body rotates about its center, so does the triangle.

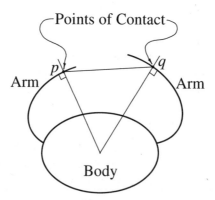

Fig. 13-1. A depiction of the body, with arms used to intercept an opponent's force at two points. The arms are drawn as arcs because, to the opponent, each point of contact *feels* like it is on the surface of an impenetrable sphere.

Note: Figure 13-1, which is drawn two-dimensionally, only shows rotation of each arm about an axis perpendicular to the page. In actual application of the principle of roundness and expansiveness just discussed, the arm must be also appropriately rotated about its axis. Aligning the surfaces both ways is necessary for deflecting the opponent's attack, three-dimensionally, in *any direction*.

Newton's Third Law

By controlling the force you exert on the opponent, you automatically control his force on you.

According to Newton's third law, if object *A* exerts a force on object *B*, then *B* exerts an equal-and-opposite force back on *A* (see Fig. 5-1). These two forces are called *an action and reaction pair*. Thus, when someone exerts force on your body with his hand, before you even do anything, your body automatically exerts a force back on his hand that is exactly equal in magnitude and opposite in direction to the force his hand exerts on your body. Similarly, when you place your hand on his body, now another two forces come into play. One is the force that you are exerting on his body with your hand. The other is the equal-and-opposite force exerted on your hand by his body. We will show how the reciprocity of action and reaction can be used in controlling and thereby neutralizing another's force on you.

Neutralizing

Shifting Off the Line of the Attack

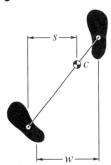

Fig. 13-2. When the weight in a 70-30 stance shifts from 70 percent on the forward foot to 100 percent on the rear foot, the center of mass *C* of the body shifts to a location over the center of the rear foot, corresponding to a sideways movement a distance *s* of approximately 80 percent of a shoulder width *w*.

Before analyzing the turning aspect of neutralization, we consider the effects of shifting the weight when in a 70-30 stance (Fig. 13-2). In fixed-stance push-hands practice, the only way to move off the line of the attack is to shift your weight (in moving-stance push-hands or in combat, there is also the option of stepping). When 70 percent of your weight is on your forward foot, your center of mass (cm) is over the line joining the centers of your feet and 70 percent of the way from the center of your rear foot to that of your front foot. When your weight shifts to 100 percent on your rear foot, your cm moves along the line joining the centers of your feet to a location directly over the center of your rear foot. It can be seen from Figure 13-2 that shifting your weight from 70 percent on your forward leg to 100 percent on your rear leg corresponds to shifting your body obliquely with a sideways component s, which is about 80 percent of a shoulder width w.

This analysis shows why sufficient width in a 70-30 stance is so important; without it, neutralization is hampered. Of course, sufficient width is also important for attaining stability and mobility.

In a self-defense situation, it may very well be necessary to step off the line of the attack.

Conclusion. When there is a committed attack to your center, just by your shifting backward in a 70-30 stance you automatically move your center off the line of attack by an amount that prevents the attack from reaching your body. In a self-defense situation, it is probably necessary to step off the line of the attack.[4]

Turning

In general, the force exerted on your body by an attacking opponent can be considered to have two components: (a) a component radially inward, directly to your center, and (b) a tangential component exerted by friction. Because the opponent should be made to feel that he is contacting a sphere that is able to rotate freely, friction is limited to only what causes the sphere (your body) to rotate. The more freely rotating your body is, the less friction is needed. Thus, the main force exerted on your body by the opponent will be essentially toward your center even if the line of the attack is *not* toward your center (Fig. 13-3).

By Newton's third law, the force exerted on the opponent by your body will be exactly equal and opposite to his force on you. Because the opponent's force will be directed toward your center, by Newton's third law, your force on him will be radially outward from your center and toward his center.

In Figure 13-3, the line of attack is off center—not because that is the way the opponent wants it to be but because you moved it off the line of the attack by shifting or stepping.

We will next use elementary physics to show how the neutralization works and the conditions under which minimum force can be used.

---

4. See video of Chen Shih-hsing (Chen Shixing) emphasizing stepping off the line in demonstrating Taiji applications (4:19–5:50): https://www.youtube.com/watch?v=uA-4gPb3tfo.

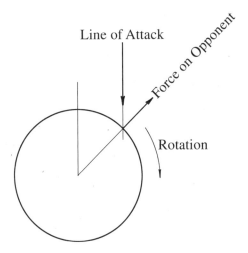

Fig. 13-3. The force of the attack on your body has two mutually perpendicular components: one is radially into your center, and the other is tangential to the (spherical) surface of your body at the point of contact. The tangential component is not shown here because it is negligibly small if your body is free to rotate.

Why Countering a Strong Attack Is Useless

If the opponent's line of attack is directly toward your center and you allow it to remain that way, the force he exerts on you can only be neutralized by an equal-and-opposite force outward from your center and back to him. Countering such a strong attack that way could require more strength than you have, resulting in your being injured. Even if you were strong enough, mounting such a defense would be ineffective because it would interfere with and stop the opponent's motion. In the words of Professor Cheng, "An opponent charges us with a force that rushes like a mighty river. What is our defense? If we attempt to confront this force head on, it will be as useless as attempting to melt iron."[5] In Taiji, the goal is to use minimal force so as not to interfere with the opponent's motion, which requires moving one's center off the line of the attack either by shifting (see Fig. 13-3) or stepping. Then the neutralizing force will be exerted at an angle to the incoming momentum. The farther your center is off the line of the attack, (a) the closer to 90 degrees the angle between the line of the attack and the line from your center to the point of contact, (b) the smaller the deflecting force needed to neutralize the attack, and (c) the less the attacker's momentum will be changed in magnitude and direction.

---

5. Cheng Man-ch'ing, *Master Cheng's Thirteen Chapters on T'ai-Chi Ch'uan*, trans. Prof. Douglas Wile (Brooklyn, NY: Sweet Ch'i Press, 1982), 31.

The Erroneous Concept of an "Incoming Force"

It is said that a force of four ounces deflects one thousand pounds.[6] What is meant by this saying is that a very powerful attack can be deflected with a very small force. Whereas its concept is very important, its wording leads to misunderstanding in explanations involving physics because it is inconsistent with Newton's third law. Namely, if A exerts a force on B, then B must exert an equal and opposite force on A. So if there is a force of one thousand pounds, it must be exerted on something (or somebody) that (or who) exerts one thousand pounds back. Here, the force that the opponent exerts would be on you, and of course you would exert an equal-and-opposite force back on him.

But the main idea is not to interact with the opponent in a way that can cause injury to yourself. The goal is to exert minimal force on the opponent and arrange that his attack clears your body. Using minimal force on the opponent means that you don't need a lot of strength. It also means that he will, by Newton's third law, use minimum force on you, which lessens the chance that you will be injured. Minimally interfering with the opponent's motion means that he will feel that he is not being thwarted, continue his motion, be more likely to overextend and, as a result, lose his balance. Then, he will either fall or pull back. If he pulls back, you can easily push or hit him.

Physics-wise, it is simply incorrect for an attack to be described in terms of an opponent's "incoming force," and therefore it is incorrect to analyze the neutralization in such terms. Maybe the opponent *intends* to exert one thousand pounds of force on you, but he is unable to do so because of how you arrange the conditions.

Whereas it is inappropriate to talk about an *incoming* force, we do need to treat the force exerted by the defender to understand the conditions for minimizing that force. Thus, in what follows, we will analyze the attack and its defense in terms of the *attacker's momentum* and the *defender's force, applied over an interval of time.*

Neutralizing with Minimum Force

In Treatise 7, Professor Cheng talks about deflecting an attack by using "no strength," which can be interpreted as decreasing the strength used to an absolute minimum (non-action). Our analysis will employ diagrams similar to those of Y. K. Chen. However, *incoming force* will be replaced by the appropriate quantity, *incoming momentum.*

A rigorous analysis would take into account that the neutralizing force changes in direction as the body turns. The analysis of the action of a changing force requires the use of vector calculus, which is beyond the scope of this

---

6. Benjamin Pang Jeng Lo, Martin Inn, Robert Amacker, and Susan Foe, eds., *The Essence of T'ai Chi Ch'uan, The Literary Tradition* (Berkeley, CA: North Atlantic Books, 1985), 37.

treatment. We will, therefore, simplify the analysis by assuming that the neutralizing force is constant in direction. The error caused by this simplification will not qualitatively affect the conclusions reached.

Because the direction of the neutralizing force is the main factor in determining its magnitude and effectiveness, our analysis must utilize quantities that have direction (thereby ruling out treating energy, which is non-directional). Momentum and force are quantities that have both magnitude and direction. Such quantities are called *vectors*.

Note: Boldface type will be used to represent vector quantities (e.g., **F**), and italics will be used to represent the magnitudes of vector quantities (e.g., F).

Because our analysis requires adding vectors, please refer to the method of doing so in Appendix 1 if necessary.

Analysis

We will next use vector addition to analyze the deflection of an incoming attack that is displaced by various amounts from a line to the defender's center. This analysis will reveal the conditions for neutralizing by using minimum force.

Momentum **P** is defined as mass times velocity and is a vector quantity because velocity has direction. Let us assume that the opponent's initial momentum is $\mathbf{P_i}$ and that the opponent's final momentum is $\mathbf{P_f}$. We will depict the defender's body as a circle (which is the cross section of a sphere). There is a principle in physics that the change in momentum $\mathbf{P_f} - \mathbf{P_i}$ equals the average force **F** multiplied by the time t during which **F** acts. Stated mathematically,

$$\mathbf{P_f} - \mathbf{P_i} = \mathbf{F} \cdot t. \qquad \text{(Eq. 1)}$$

Force has magnitude and direction and, therefore, must be treated as a vector quantity. As mentioned earlier, a force radially outward from a rotating sphere would be changing both in magnitude and direction, so, to simplify things, we will assume here that the force remains constant. The result of this force is to change the direction of the momentum to be tangent to the sphere (deflected harmlessly away from the body).

From Eq. 1, above, it can be seen that the force used for deflecting the opponent's incoming momentum is minimized (the legendary use of four ounces) if the time to do it is prolonged and if the opponent's change in momentum $\mathbf{P_f} - \mathbf{P_i}$ is kept small (only a small sideways deflection, just large enough to cause the attack to clear your body).

Inverting Eq. 1, we get

$$\mathbf{P_f} = \mathbf{P_i} + \mathbf{F} \cdot t.$$

See Figure 13-4 for the application of the above vector equation for the force required for deflecting incoming momentum displaced different amounts from the center of the defender.

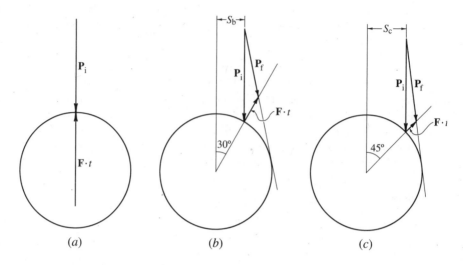

(a) (b) (c)

Fig. 13-4. (a) P_i is radially inward. Therefore $F \bullet t$ is equal and opposite to P_i, and P_f is zero. (b) Center has shifted to the left by S_b. P_i is directed at a 30-degree angle to a line drawn from the center to the point of contact. Therefore the line of $F \bullet t$ makes a 30-degree angle to that of P_i. P_f is tangent to the circle and smaller in magnitude than P_i, and the magnitude of $F \bullet t$ is much smaller than that of P_i. (c) Center has shifted to the left by S_c. P_i, is directed at a 45-degree angle to the radius. Therefore the line of $F \bullet t$ makes a 45-degree angle to that of P_i. P_f is tangent to the circle and slightly smaller in magnitude than P_i, and the magnitude of $F \bullet t$ is even smaller than when P_i is directed at a 30-degree angle to the radius.

Conclusion. With reference to Figure 13-4, as the angle between P_i and the radius approaches 90 degrees, the magnitude of $F \bullet t$ approaches zero, and P_f approaches P_i. *Thus, the more you can move your center off the line of your opponent's attack, the smaller the deflecting force needed and the smaller the change in the opponent's momentum.* Also, the longer the amount of time t that your force is exerted, the less your force needs to be. As a result, you are not harmed, you use minimum force, and the opponent's motion is almost unchanged, which disrupts his balance.

The Reason Your Deflecting Force Should Be Radially Outward from Your Center

It can now be explained why in neutralizing, your force must be radially out from your center. Imagine that instead, you were to exert a tangential component of force on the opponent. From the middle diagram in Figure 13-4, it can be seen that you would then interact with the opponent's incoming momentum in such a way that he no longer would feel as though he is contacting a freely rotating sphere but one that requires force to turn. That resistance would likely alert the opponent, who would change his attack.

Next, again imagine that instead of exerting force on your opponent radially outward from your center, you were to add a tangential component of force away from the opponent. From the middle diagram in Figure 13-4, it can be seen that the effect would be to interact with the opponent's incoming momentum in such a way that he no longer feels as though he is contacting a freely rotating sphere but one that turns faster than it should and pulls him. Whereas pulling the opponent is a valuable tactic, it can only be done effectively *after* the opponent's attack is neutralized. Again, the opponent would likely be alerted by this inconsistent rotational rate and change his attack.

Thus, it can be seen that the success of the neutralization requires that you exert force radially outward from your center. Adding a component of force in any other direction is counterproductive or wasteful.

Next, consider what happens when the surface presented to the opponent is not perpendicular to the line from your center to that surface. In this case, the surface automatically exerts a component of force that is not radially outward from your center. The only way to lessen this force is to withdraw the surface rather than turn your body. The result is that the opponent can follow the change and end up catching you, in which case you have not neutralized but unsuccessfully run away. This analysis illustrates the importance of keeping the surface of your body, at the point of contact with the opponent, perpendicular to the line drawn from your center to that point.

Attacking

Your attack must be directly from your center to that of the opponent. If your attack is not from your center, the reaction to it will cause your body to rotate, thereby dissipating the energy of the attack. Moreover, if the attack is not to the center of the opponent, it will cause the opponent's body to rotate, thereby neutralizing the force of the attack. It is very important to establish a line from your center to that of the opponent before attacking.

Yearning K. Chen's Alternative Way of Deflecting an Attack

Yearning K. Chen was an inside student of Yang Cheng-fu. Chen's book on Taiji includes a chapter, "Taiji as Related to Dynamics."[7] In that chapter, Chen analyzes several cases of an opponent's 120-pound "incoming force" directed toward the defender's center. In each case the defender strikes the attacker with a 60-pound force radially-outward from his center at a particular angle to the direction of the attack. Figures 13-5 and 13-6 depict two of the six cases shown in Chen's book.

The idea is that the defender's strike, if correctly timed, causes the direction of the attacker's motion to change sideways, thereby disrupting his balance. Thus, he is injured by the strike or susceptible to being struck while in a weakened state.

Whereas Chen's analysis appears to be inconsistent physics-wise, its intended concept is valuable and definitely worthy of consideration and clarification.

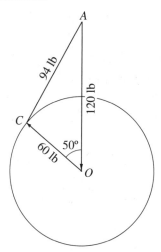

Fig. 13-5. A sketch of part of the diagram in Y. K. Chen's book in which *AO* is an attacker's "incoming" 120-pound force, and *OC* is a 60-pound force exerted by the defender. The result shown is that the attacker now has a 94-pound "incoming force" in an unexpected direction.

If the angle is greater than 90 degrees (shown in Fig. 13-6), then the striking force pulls the attacker off balance to the side and increases his motion.

---

7. Yearning K. Chen, *Tai-Chi Chuan: Its Effects and Practical Applications*, 15–17.

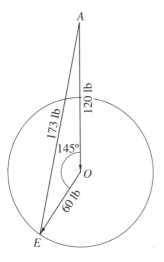

Fig. 13-6. A sketch of part of the diagram in Y. K. Chen's book in which *AO* is an attacker's "incoming" 120-pound force, and *OE* is a 60-pound force exerted by the defender. The result shown is that the attacker now has a 173-pound "incoming force" in an unexpected direction.

The inconsistency in each of Figures 13-5 and 13-6 appears to be that the attacker's and defender's forces are *unequal* in amount, and they are not opposite in direction, thereby violating Newton's third law. Namely, any force exerted by the attacker must have the *same* magnitude as that exerted by the defender and be *opposite* in direction. And there can't be a force that doesn't have such a reaction. Also, it is only meaningful to add forces that are on the same object, and they are not so here.

Clarification of Yearning K. Chen 's Analysis of Deflecting an Attack

Here is an interpretation of Chen's analysis that is consistent with Newton's third law: in order for the attacker to exert a striking force of 120 pounds on you, he must mobilize his body to be in balance at the moment of impact. If the attack succeeds, at that moment there will be a reaction force of 120 pounds on him exerted by you. For his body to be in balance at that moment, he must simultaneously exert a countering force of 120 pounds backward on the ground, the reaction to which is a forward balancing force of 120 pounds on him. If at the moment of his expected strike, you strike him with a force of 60 pounds at an angle with the attacking direction, it will add to the forward force of 120 pounds that the ground exerts on him. The resultant force (the sum of those two forces) will then be in a new direction and not have anything to balance it because the attacker will have failed to hit you. Thus, the attacker will lose balance and fall or will have been injured by your strike.

So in Figure 13-5, all forces shown are on the attacker, and the resultant force on him has a magnitude of 94 pounds, and that force should be directed from *A* to *C* (the direction of the 94-pound force is absent from Chen's diagram). A similar statement holds for Figure 13-6.

Chen's idea is to use disrupting and possibly damaging force on the opponent rather than moving aside, causing him to fall into emptiness, which is another option he mentions.

In Conclusion

When I studied with Cheng Man-ch'ing in the early 1970s, he greatly emphasized the importance of neutralization in push-hands practice. He felt that we should not push each other with any power until we learned how to neutralize. That way, the person being pushed would have a better chance of success in learning to neutralize. At that time, few (if any) of us were able to neutralize. It was not until years after Professor Cheng's death that his *Thirteen Treatises*, written in Chinese in 1946, was translated into English. Had that book been available in English when Professor Cheng was alive, I am sure that we would have had many questions for him about Treatise 7. As a result, we might have made much faster progress in learning to neutralize.

It is interesting that two native Chinese students of Yang Cheng-fu—Cheng Man-ch'ing, born over a century ago, and Yearning K. Chen—considered physics to be a useful tool in explaining neutralization. Practicing intuitively for many years in an effort to master an art is certainly of great value. However, using every tool—in this case physics—cannot but hasten mastery for some and can make the difference between partial expertise and mastery for others.

Chapter 14

Non-Intention, Intention, and "a Hand Is Not a Hand"

Non-Intention

Non-intention is a Taiji principle that can be quite perplexing. Non-intention implies that while doing an action, there is no conscious thought of the goal of that action and no conscious determination to accomplish that goal. By comparison, being-in-the-moment implies that in any action, the mind is appropriately and totally involved in that action, with no excursions into the past or future. Even though they might seem to be unrelated, the principles of being in the moment and non-intention are similar and complementary.

It is natural to wonder how one can accomplish anything without a goal, a desire to accomplish that goal, or looking into the past or future. It would seem that in a self-defense situation, it would be necessary to have the intention to win out, act with the right timing and skill resulting from one's training, be aware of future possibilities, and weigh those possibilities against what has happened before.

Here is where the distinction between conscious and subconscious minds is useful. Whereas the observational aspect of the conscious mind is disrupted by contemplating winning or being preoccupied with an awareness of all of the future possibilities in a situation, the subconscious mind can encompass those possibilities. The conscious mind merely observes through the senses and augments what is being accomplished by the subconscious mind, moment by moment.

Seeing action as guided mainly by the subconscious mind is the key to understanding non-intention and being in the moment. That is, with correct training and repeated practice, you need not have conscious intention or be conscious of the past or future—your subconscious mind takes care of that.

When your conscious mind attempts to deal with, for example, what comes next, it is not in the moment but making an excursion into the future. When your conscious mind moves into the future, the present passes by. Now your conscious mind is disadvantageously in the past, and you are behind, thereby sacrificing success. Moreover, when your conscious mind deals with what comes next, it is usurping your subconscious mind's role, and it is incapable of fulfilling that role in a timely fashion because that role involves too many actions and references to the past and future.

So non-intention and being in the moment require that the conscious mind is appropriately involved in overseeing events as they unfold.

Additionally, when you have a conscious intention to do something in a physical confrontation, an opponent can easily pick up that intention and use it to his or her advantage. Also, when your conscious mind momentarily shifts from the present, a trained opponent can pick that up too and immediately seize the advantage.

The Mental Transmission of Intention

One of the basic concepts in internal martial arts is that a skilled opponent can "read" our intentions and, thereby, be ready to thwart our attack or defense. Once there is a connection between two people, if trained, one of them can read the intention of the other directly, even without any input to the conventionally named senses (visual, auditory, tactile, etc.).

Ninjutsu, which I studied with Kevin Harrington and Michael DeMaio, is a Japanese art whose principles have much in common with those of Taijiquan. In that art, the mental projection of intention to harm another is called *sakki*, translated as *the force of the killer*[1] (see characters in Fig. 14-1, and compare with that in Fig. 14-2). An important part of Ninja training is to develop the ability to perceive and respond to *sakki*. The goal is to be protected from another's attack by moving to safety at the right instant—even when the attacker is not seen!

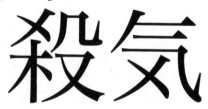

Fig. 14-1. The characters for the Japanese word, *sakki*. The character on the left is *satsu*, which means *kill*. The character on the right is *ki*, which is essentially the same as *qi* in Chinese (see Fig. 14-2). So *sakki* refers to the "intent" of the killer.[2]

1. Stephen K. Hayes, *The Ninja and Their Secret Fighting Art* (Rutland, VT: Charles E. Tuttle Company, 1981), 144–148.
2. See Andrew N. Nelson, *The Modern Reader's Japanese-English Character Dictionary: Original Classic* (North Clarendon, VT: Tuttle Publishing, 1995), 524.

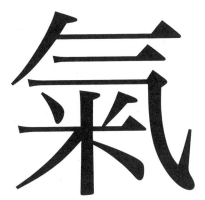

Fig. 14-2. The Chinese character for *qi*. The bottom part represents rice (simplified in Fig. 14-1 as a cross), and the top part represents steam.

The following seemingly paradoxical quote from the Taiji Classics may refer to the ability of a skilled practitioner to sense the intention of an opponent to attack:

> It is said, "If others don't move, I don't move. If others move slightly, I move first."[3]

> —Wu Yu-hsiang

Whereas in most self-defense situations it is important not to have intention, intention can be actively used to freeze, startle, or distract an opponent to provide time to escape to safety or to move him to a position more beneficial for attacking him. In Ninja training, however, intention is often purposely used to enable a training partner to sense and properly utilize another's intention.

---

3. Benjamin Pang Jeng Lo, Martin Inn, Robert Amacker, and Susan Foe, eds., *The Essence of T'ai Chi Ch'uan, The Literary Tradition* (Berkeley, CA: North Atlantic Books, 1985), 57.

Learning to Sense *Sakki*

Experiment 14-1. The most basic element of experiencing and responding to *sakki* can be practiced by two people as follows: Person *A* (the "attacker") stands behind person *B*. *A* holds a relatively harmless model knife. *A* then imagines cutting *B* with his knife. In order for the imagined attack to be realistic, *A* must have the intention to do harm even though no harm will ensue. When *B* feels the urgency to move away from the attack, he or she turns around. If *B* does not feel the attack after a reasonable amount of time, *A* "cuts" *B*. That way the victim can then review what he or she experienced during the stages of being threatened and learn to recognize those feelings when they occur again.

The roles of *A* and *B* should be alternately exchanged.

Often, beginners who do the above exercise fail to consciously recognize the feeling of being in danger, but their bodies "know" and react by moving visibly. It does not take long, however, for beginners to recognize the urgent feeling of *sakki*.

With continued practice, it is possible to feel the part of the body under attack and move at the right instant. Eventually, the analytical mind is not needed; the intention of an opponent will result in the Ninja automatically moving to safety.

Testing *Sakki* Sensitivity and Timing of Movement to Safety

In Ninjutsu, the *godan* test (the test for fifth-degree black belt) requires the applicant to sit on the floor in *seiza*, which means sitting correctly, with knees together, back straight, and buttocks resting on heels. Grandmaster Masaaki Hatsumi stands behind the applicant. He holds a *shinai* (a "sword" made from bamboo strips that make a loud sound on impact but don't cause injury) over his head, "blade" extending backward, ready to "cut." Suddenly and with great intention and speed, Hatsumi swings the *shinai* downward on the applicant's head. The belt is awarded only if the applicant moves at the right time (see video[4] and another video[5]). If the applicant moves too early (before Hatsumi's action is committed), Hatsumi can easily change and hit the applicant, and if the applicant moves too late, he or she will of course also get hit.

Note in the linked videos the strong intention evidenced in Grandmaster Hatsumi's face just as he swings the *shinai*. At that moment but not before, he

---

4. https://www.youtube.com/watch?v=-zNP7-unHrw.
5. https://www.youtube.com/watch?v=i-GidagO6C8.

is generating in himself the intention to do severe physical harm, at the same time subconsciously knowing that the applicant will not be injured if he or she fails the test.

Most of the applicants in the first video are feeling Hatsumi's intention but moving prematurely. At one point, Hatsumi exclaims, "Very good. Excellent," because the applicant is feeling the initiation of his thought to start the sword motion. Nevertheless, that applicant's analytical mind gets in the way, and he moves prematurely, thus failing the test.

Whereas a highly trained opponent can know our intention without any visual, auditory, or tactile cues, almost any opponent will know our intention if these cues are physically evident. Thus, we train to contact an opponent softly and move with unification and continuity. However, even a shift of weight or the shape of a hand telegraphs information that can be "read" about our intention. That is why a weapon or even a fist is usually not shown before its use, and the weighting of stances and transitions is so important.

Wild animals have a much greater ability than that of humans to perceive danger or respond to a connection initiated by another being. If they did not, they would not stay alive very long. But in my experience, humans, too, possess this ability and can vastly increase it.

"A Hand Is Not a Hand"

When I had been studying with Cheng Man-ch'ing for a few years, he said in class, "A hand is not a hand—every part of the body is a hand, but hands have nothing to do with it." By then, I had become accustomed to this type of paradoxical statement. Whereas I had no idea what it meant, I knew that it must be meaningful and important. However, the understanding of a concept in Taiji sometimes occurs a long time after exposure to it.

"The Beauteous Hand" and "Setting the Wrist"

Professor Cheng also emphasized what he called "the beauteous hand" (Fig. 14-3), which means allowing the fingers and wrists to attain their most centered, relaxed, and natural alignment. He claimed that doing so enabled *qi* to reach the tips of the fingers. It should be noted that Cheng's teacher, Yang Cheng-fu, emphasized "setting the wrist"[6] of the potentially striking hand at the end of each movement, which meant bending the wrist so that the palm faced forward. Yang's purpose[7] of setting the wrist was to expand the palm by using nei jin rather than by contraction of the forearm muscles. Yang was

---

6. Some use the words *settling* or *seating* the wrist.

7. Fu Zhongwen, *Mastering Yang-Style Taijiquan*, trans. Louis Swaim (Berkeley, CA: Blue Snake Books, 2006), 29.

highly skilled. His wrists were so relaxed and pliable that he was able to bend them by expansion beyond what others can do that way. Professor Cheng retained setting the wrists in the "Beginning" movement and did so subtly in other movements.[89]

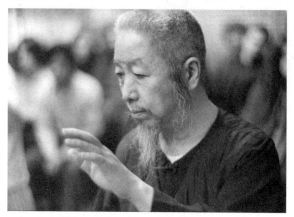

Fig. 14-3. Cheng Man-ch'ing's "beauteous hand."[10]

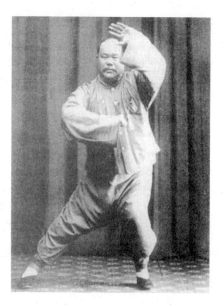

Fig. 14-4. Yang Cheng-fu in the transition "Turn and Chop with Fist."

8. See https://www.youtube.com/watch?v=3_BKwlpOAkk&t=101s.

9. Some use the words *settling* or *seating* the wrist.

10. Photo by Ken Van Sickle.

Differences between Yang and Cheng styles are treated in the author's Internet article cited in the footnote below.[11] As is often the case, there can be two (or more) correct ways of doing something. However, some photos of Yang reveal his wrists to be beautifully neutral during transitions (Fig. 14-4).

It took some time for me to realize that "a hand is not a hand" and "the beauteous hand" encompass health, self-development, and self-defense aspects. They promote recognizing and releasing contractive strength and cultivating the flow of *qi*, and they illustrate the principles of non-action, non-intention, non-attachment, being in the moment, and unification of all parts of the body.

Why Are Hands So Important?

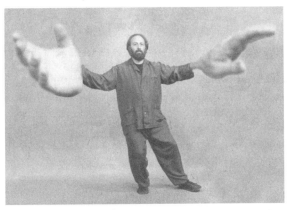

Fig. 14-5. A *Sensory Homunculus*, which is a model of a human body, with the size of each part proportional to its sensory connections to the cortex of a human brain. This figure was roughly created by the author, using an old photograph of himself and an old version of Photoshop®. A *Motor Homunculus*, for which the size of each is part proportional to its motor connections to the cortex of a human brain, would be similar.

Our hands have many more sensory and motor nerve endings than other parts of our bodies (see Fig. 14-5). As a consequence, our thoughts are readily expressed through our hands. When you touch another person, the pressure and movement of your hand tells that person your intention. Moreover, by learning not to put any intention in the hands (by allowing a natural, centered shape), you are training not only the physical aspect of non-intention but also its corresponding mental state.

---

11. For occurrences and comparisons of movements in both the Yang and Cheng Man-ch'ing forms, visit https://www.chuckrowtaichi.com/CMCvsYang.html.

Hands and Non-Intention

Physically, "a hand is not a hand" means that when your hand touches the opponent, it does not act, feel, or move like a hand. Everyone knows what hands and fingers can do—block, punch, pull, push, deflect, stab, poke, pinch, slap, and grasp limbs, fingers, skin, neck, hair, etc. But the trunk of the body can do little to attack and is vulnerable. So when a hand feels, moves, and acts like a hand, the opponent becomes alerted, ready to change, and ready to take defensive or offensive action. If, however, your arms and hands are so thoroughly unified with the body that they act and feel to the opponent like an extension of the trunk of your body, they are not threatening. That is, during neutralization, when your arms and hands lead the opponent off your center, it should feel to him that he contacted your body, not your arm or hand. And that point of contact moves, not with any intention of yours but seemingly passively, as a result of his action. That is why, in doing the Taiji form, it is important for the shape of the hands to be natural and their movement to be as much as possible a result of the unified turning and shifting of the body. Moreover, there should not be any mental state of intention in a self-defense situation except at the instant that a strike or kick contacts the opponent. At that instant, intention is crucial.

Corollary: An elbow is not an elbow, and a foot is not a foot. The same idea applies to any part of the body.

Experiment 14-2. Caution: For this experiment, you will need a partner who is very controlled because squeezing the carotid arteries (one on each side of your neck) can cause loss of consciousness in about fifteen seconds, with possible serious aftereffects.

In this scenario, the opponent, who is facing you, succeeds in grabbing your neck with both hands, strangling you. A reaction by an untrained person might be to grab both wrists and try to pry his hands off. Try doing that action with your partner, and feel how it causes an immediate increase in the strength of the hold. Instead, just gently touch each wrist with a hand, and move your whole body backward without moving your hands (as in the movement "Withdraw and Push"). The constraint here is that your hands do not move even though every other part of your body does. I learned this application from the late Lou Kleinsmith, a senior student of Professor Cheng.

The Transmission of Intention Over a Distance

The Transmission of *Qi* in Healing

Intentionally "sending" healing "energy" to another person can be thought of as the constructive counterpart of *sakki*. The word *sending* is in quotes because it is not clear that anything is really sent. The word *energy* is also in quotes because, scientifically, that word may not apply.

It is generally accepted by Qigong (and Reiki) healers that *qi* (*ki*) of one person can beneficially affect another even over many miles, and my own experience is consistent with that idea. However, there is no formal scientific acceptance that the *qi* of one person can be transmitted to another even when the individuals are in visual proximity—let alone when they are miles apart. Certainly, present science has not uncovered any mechanism by which such a distant effect might occur.

Currently there is scientific research and tentative acceptance that when seeing a person doing an action, your own bioelectricity is sympathetically activated for initiating that action. Such scientific study is, however, in its infancy.

How Can Intention and *Qi* Be Transmitted?

Some experimentation has been done with the distant effects of intention, and it is thought that quantum effects may be involved. Whereas *qi* may involve production of electromagnetic phenomena external to the "sender's" body, as the separation of individuals involved increases from very close, any such fields would die off rapidly. So it is unlikely that electromagnetic fields could have an effect at distances of more than several feet.

Perhaps the underlying phenomenon involves the interaction of physical quantities[12] that are known but which scientists have been unable to measure.[13] Or, it may involve physical quantities that are not yet known. Perhaps the mode of transmission is not even physical, in which case, science in its present form may not have the tools with which to uncover the process involved.

"Empty Force"

Empty force refers to the idea that one person can cause another to do specific movements when the two are a distance apart. There are Internet videos

---

12. A physical quantity is the property of a phenomenon, body, or substance, that can be quantified by measurement. (See http://en.wikipedia.org/wiki/Physical_quantity/.) Some examples are length, mass, time, and speed.

13. The following is an example of a phenomenon that involves the interaction of known physical quantities but which scientists are currently unable to measure: theoretically, when an elevator filled with occupants descends, the earth moves a corresponding amount in the opposite direction. Because the mass of the earth is so much greater than that of the elevator, the movement of the earth is far too small to be measured.

showing a teacher causing his students to move seemingly uncontrollably, writhing on the floor unable to rise, and even appearing to be in pain. And the teacher accomplishes this feat without a touch. Other videos show the same teacher unable to affect certain challengers, who just stand there, unmoved and apparently unaffected.

One explanation may be that, similar to *sakki* training, empty-force training is a tool that prepares students to become sensitive to the negative intention of another and to respond accordingly. The resulting sensitivity then enables them to be more able to move to safety. However, those who are untrained probably will not be affected, and empty force may not stop a determined attacker. But that doesn't mean that the basic principle is invalid.

Author's View

I have come to accept that a sentient being can influence the bioelectrical impulses or other internal conditions of others even when the external actions of that being cannot be perceived by the known senses (sight, hearing, pressure, etc.) of the others. Of course, for such effects to occur, a connection needs to be established, and there must be receptivity on the part of the others. Perhaps additional conditions may be required.

I have adopted the idea that, instead of thinking that I am "sending" healing *qi* to another person, I am just intensifying my *qi* for assisting that person's *self-healing*. I view a recipient as activating and intensifying his or her own healing apparatus—even at a distance. That view has the fortuitous implication that nothing of mine is being expended when I am doing healing on another. Thus, I can just intensify my own *qi* without becoming drained or taking on the subject's symptoms. Also, my ego is much less involved because I am not the one doing the healing; I am merely a facilitator. Additionally, I benefit from the intensification of my own *qi* and the exhilaration of knowing that someone has similarly benefited.

Chapter 15
Maximizing Your Progress
in Taiji

"Petit à petit l'oiseau fait son nid."
Translation: *"Little by little, the bird builds its nest."*

Studying Taiji

Practice

It is important for those who have attended classes in Yoga, Pilates, aerobics, and other popular exercises to understand that Taiji is different. Attending Taiji class is necessary but not sufficient—consistent, daily practice is required. Without practice, not only is little or no progress made, achieving the benefits is almost impossible (see the Chinese characters for *study* in Fig. 15-1) and the explanation below.

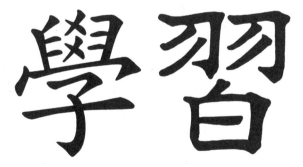

Fig. 15-1. The Chinese characters for the word *xuéxí*. The first character, *xué* (*learn*), shows a child with a dome above it to protect it. Above the dome are two helping hands, and the *x*'s represent the child's immature attempts at writing. The second character, *xí* (*practice*), shows wings above a rectangular character which is thought to be a corruption

of the character for *self* (an extra horizontal line is missing). The meaning is that the bird must learn to fly by itself. So studying involves first being helped to learn (*yin* aspect), but then you must practice (*yang* aspect).

Many—especially those who learn very quickly—are used to getting things fast without doing any work. That attribute works for certain studies but not for Taiji. Just missing one day of practice causes much to evaporate. Thus, it is suggested that a student should not go to bed without having practiced that day, and practicing twice daily is far preferable.

Fear of Making Mistakes

Some students avoid practicing because they worry about making mistakes. Actually, making mistakes is *necessary* for learning and progressing at Taiji. In school, we were taught not to make mistakes because we were being trained to work on an assembly line, where mistakes slow production. True learning, however, requires mistake-making.

For example, when you initiate an erroneous computer command, you learn not to do that again. But sometimes, you also discover a useful tool you never knew existed. Mistakes are valuable learning tools.

Obstacles to Learning Taiji

It has been suggested that a room full of monkeys typing randomly would eventually reproduce the works of Shakespeare. But the time required would in all probability be greater than that of the age of the universe.[1]

Trying to truly master Taiji can be similar to the monkeys on the typewriters. There are many books, videos, and websites devoted to Taiji. There are also many teachers of varying skill levels, teaching abilities, and willingness to impart their knowledge.

Whereas confusion, plateaus, frustrations, and contradictions are part of studying any art, such difficulties especially apply to Taiji. Many obstacles result not only from the historic family nature of Taiji as a martial art but also from bewildering transmission, whether intended (for secrecy) or not. These issues are discussed next.

The Historical Family Nature of Taiji

Over much of martial-arts history, there have been inner students and outsiders. Outsiders were taught but seldom given the full art. Inner students were almost always family members of true masters and usually started learning as children. Their close contact with masters at a young age and thereafter enabled them to learn in a way outsiders could not. Thus, most of us

---

1. See https://en.wikipedia.org/wiki/Infinite_monkey_theorem.

who do not have the privilege of learning in such a manner must endeavor to make up for this lack creatively, by using every possible tool.

Secrecy

Taijiquan (*quan* = *fist*) was historically a martial art. A hundred years ago in China, knowing a martial art could mean the difference between life and death. Thus, if the wrong outsiders learned it, they could then become a deadly threat to their teacher. So Taijiquan was kept secret for a long time. As a result, there are few left who were exposed to a full teaching or are able to transmit it.

Occasionally, an outsider who was trusted and showed high potential might be adopted and then treated as an inner student. An example is Yang Lu-chan's adoption by the Chen family.

The historical reason for not freely teaching outsiders no longer exists. Today, knowledge of hand-to-hand combat for self-protection is not essential in many regions and has become mostly obsolete in war. And Taiji is now done mostly for health and self-development.

Even for those who were given the inner teaching and want to share it, centuries-old customs tend to persist and are hard to break. The old secretive ways are so ingrained that those who have the knowledge find it hard to part with it. So students must lift themselves up by their own bootstraps in order to progress. Unless you are fortunate enough to have been provided an inner teaching, it is necessary to rely on tools of learning beyond coming to class regularly, practicing assiduously, and fully using your creative faculties for understanding.

Ways That Teachers Teach Beginners

It should be realized that teachers strive to do their best but may be subject to the following considerations:

1. They may teach like their teachers did/do, out of respect.
2. They may teach simplistically so that more students can get it ("paint-by-numbers" Taiji).
3. They may eliminate elements that are too advanced for most students to learn and for which teaching them would squander valuable class time.
4. They may eliminate important elements that their teachers warned them to keep secret.
5. They may eliminate what they were taught but don't sufficiently understand.
6. They may eliminate what they understand and can do but are unable to properly explain (language-skill limitations or lack of teaching experience).

7. They may emphasize *qi* connections and easily remembered landmarks ("Kodak" moments). The result might be that students incorrectly stop their movement at these places.

Students must understand such teaching considerations and generate their own ways of transcending them.

Dealing with Obstacles

Cultivating the Persistence of Your Expectation

When you see those who are highly skilled, there is a tendency to think they were born with that skill, and you tend not to realize that they had to put in a lot of work to achieve what they can do. However, if no students surpass their teacher(s), those arts and their associated wisdom severely deteriorate over time.

Over the decades that I have taught physics, I have observed that often students sabotage their learning process by thinking, "I'll never be able to do that." Expressing such an idea—or just thinking it—programs your subconscious mind to blindly accept the impossibility of succeeding. The door is then closed to any possibility of achieving a desired benefit. Henry Ford (1863–1947) aptly said:

> Whether you think you can or you think you can't, you're right.

Abstaining from negative thinking does not mean that you should go to the other extreme. Just see things as they are, and understand that things of great value take time to achieve. Allow your skill level to evolve naturally.

Use All of Your Tools

Students of any Teaching often lack the tools to make refinements to what they learn. Such a process requires critical thinking, analytical skills, perseverance, and knowledge of other arts such as science, mathematics, philosophy, etc. Ford also said:

> If you need a machine [or tool] and don't buy it, then you will ultimately find that you have paid for it and [still] don't have it.

A similar truth holds for tools for learning Taiji. Of course, excelling at Taiji requires consistent practice. But having and utilizing the proper tool is essential for getting any job done efficiently, and a price is paid for not doing so. But once you have that tool, its usefulness will carry through to new and seemingly unrelated material.

Tools of Learning

Tools for learning include the Internet, videos, books, workshops, group practice, reflection, visualization, dreams, lots of experimentation, and having an appropriate succession of teachers of Taiji and related arts such as Qigong, healing, and meditation. Another important tool is periodic reference to the Taiji principles, the primary ones of which are non-action, being in the moment, circularity, continuity, naturalness, balance of *yin* and *yang*, non-attachment, non-intention, *song*, and the cultivation of *nei jin* (expansive strength).

In my view, additional powerful tools for understanding movement arts such as Taiji are physics, anatomy, physiology, mathematics, psychology, and others listed below.

Physics is the study of stability, strength, and movement through an understanding of force; leverage; stable, unstable, and neutral equilibrium; friction; pressure; linear momentum; inertia; kinetic energy; potential energy; gravity; center of mass; straight-line and circular motion; speed; acceleration; angular momentum; wave and periodic motion; hydrostatics; hydrodynamics; elasticity; and tensile, torsional, shear, and compressional stresses.

Anatomy involves an understanding of muscles, ligaments, tendons, and optimal alignment of bones.

Physiology involves an understanding of the organs, breathing, and the circulatory, neurological, hormonal, eliminative, immune, and balance systems.

Mathematics helps us with an understanding of spatial relations, axes, planes, angles, vectors, and perspective.

Psychology sheds light on conscious and unconscious thought, learning, perception and perceptual illusions, memory, and brain function.

Philosophy provides tools for analyzing and clarifying complex ideas.

Intuition is an important but much-neglected aspect of Taiji training. Intuition steers students to their ideal teachers, guides their interactions with teachers, and helps them to benefit from their teachers' modalities. Intuition also helps you know when to change teachers should that be appropriate.

Writing is of tremendous value. When I studied with William C. C. Ch'en in the 1970s and 1980s, I often took notes. For some reason my note-taking annoyed my classmates. When Ch'en sensed their reaction, he said to me directly, "Take your time, That's good." My interpretation was that he was also telling my classmates that they might do likewise.

One of the values in writing things down is that you are forced thereby to clarify your thinking. Another value is that you tend to emblazon the content of what you write on your mind. Moreover, your written record is something to which you can refer should your memory evaporate. I still have all of my class notes from all of my martial arts teachers and often refer back to them. A valuable byproduct is seeing your progress and increase in understanding.

Experimentation is essential in order to progress in any endeavor. As we go on, we tend to become captured and fixated on what we have learned at an early stage and find those concepts and tools very difficult to set aside in favor of something more appropriate and valuable. Just as we constantly need to remind ourselves to let go of habitual, unnecessary muscular tension, we also need to periodically reevaluate what is firmly embedded in our conceptual framework. Doing so is in keeping with the Buddhist idea of "seeing things as they are" and "non-attachment."

As beginners, we were taught simple ways of remembering the movements. For example, "holding a ball" in "Ward Off Left," and "left palm-up under right elbow" in "Roll Back" are firmly emblazoned in the minds of all of Professor Cheng's progeny. Freezing what should be "Kodak" moments, however, tends to be at the expense of recognizing the essential elements of the movements. These elements would otherwise reveal themselves if allowed to do so. Instead of holding onto what was learned in "kindergarten," it is extremely valuable to put those items in your back pocket and try doing movements in such a way that the feeling of the movements becomes a teaching tool.

Accessing the appropriate source of knowledge can substantially accelerate your progress. Sources can be books, videos, the Internet, teachers, classmates, and your students (if you are teaching). As a student, it is crucial to listen to others' questions and the teacher's answers.

Ask yourself and others questions. Asking others questions not only helps you, it can also help them. Teachers especially love questions, which add to their knowledge, teaching repertoire, and exhilaration. Even when the same question is asked twice in a row, an experienced teacher will provide a second answer introducing an important, new dimension. Asking a carefully formulated question at the right time can lead to a pivotal moment in your progress. Always seek an answer based on the Taiji principles or other appropriate branches of knowledge.

Visualization is an important tool that requires only mental energy and time and can be done while sitting or even lying in bed. Visualization provides dividends beyond that of learning the material at hand. Dividends include improvement in memory and observational and learning skills. Also, by visualizing a movement without doing it outwardly, baggage of unnatural, habitual movement can be reduced.

Knowing your limitations and adjusting to them is important and totally in keeping with the spirit of Taiji. Limitations can be injuries, pain, or lack of strength, mobility, or range of motion. Rather than ignoring or masking pain, it is important to recognize that pain provides a feedback system, which, if utilized, can facilitate its reduction or even promote healing. For example, there is great therapeutic value in doing movement that would normally produce pain but doing it in a way that avoids it by "sneaking" through without pain. Practicing movement that way educates your everyday way of moving to be less likely to produce or exacerbate an injury.

One way of taking limitations into account is in altering Taiji movements subtly and appropriately, based on your limitations or those of your students. A possible example is the difference between the current and earlier Yang style as taught by Yang Cheng-fu, specifically, that of the inward turning of the rear foot. In the earlier version, to which Cheng Man-ch'ing and his classmates appear to have been exposed, when transitioning from one posture to another, the rear foot remains at 90 degrees during stepping with the other foot and turns 45 degrees inward at the end of the movement. The current way, as evidently taught by Yang in his later years, involves presetting the rear foot 45 degrees inward *prior* to stepping with the other foot.[2] It is much harder to step 90 degrees than 45 degrees. In his later years, Yang might have changed that feature because of his own or his students' knee or other problems.

Summary
Throughout this book, I have endeavored to involve the use of the above tools—including even metaphysics where applicable. Whereas these tools are not the be-all or end-all, they are extremely useful. Unfortunately, they are insufficiently applied to Taiji movement. Instead, gobbledygook and mystical concepts are preferred by some over science, which they disparage!

Dangers of Overusing Images in Movement Arts
Images (imagining that which is not present or actual) are very helpful and are used in many movement arts such as dance, Yoga, acting, sports, and Taiji. Such images are provided to beginners so that they can have something to remember and practice. However, imagery is only a tool, which can become problematic when used beyond a certain point.

An example of an image used in Taiji is the idea of "swimming on land," which involves doing the Taiji movements while imagining the air to have the consistency and resistance of water. After continued practice, the air is said to feel like iron (see Chapter 3). Other Taiji examples are imagining holding a ball, imagining your head suspended from above, and imagining your center of gravity to be far below the ground.

The problem is that imagining something untrue involves self-deception. Then, sustaining the state provided by the image past its usefulness requires continuing that deception, which is limiting to our understanding and becomes inefficient because it requires the continued, unnecessary use of the conscious mind. The conscious mind is slow and can only encompass a few things at a time. Instead of unnecessarily burdening the conscious mind, it is better to see things as they are; namely, just learn how to achieve the benefit suggested by the image but without any prolonged need for it. Then the

---

2. See https://www.chuckrowtaichi.com/CMCvsYang.html for comparisons of movements in both the Yang and Cheng Man-ch'ing forms.

subconscious mind, which can deal with myriad tasks simultaneously, can take over, and you can *own the principle* instead of having to rely on a limiting and incomplete artifice.

Using an image beyond its usefulness also involves a preconception and violates the principles of non-intention and being in the moment (see Chapter 15). Being attached to an image then masks sensory input and creates an obstacle to ever getting past the image and going to the next level.

Consider the image of holding a ball between the palms of the hands. This image is useful in remembering landmarks within the movements and also helps students recognize the sensation of a *qi*-induced state. Students initially taught this image tend to use it even when they become advanced in their practice. The result is that, instead of experiencing the natural swing and continuity of circular motion of their arms in doing such moves as "Ward Off Left," they *reach* for an imaginary ball with their hands. Having that intention involves being in the future instead of in the moment and disrupts what would otherwise be a natural flow.

Another image provided beginners is that of holding a raw egg under your arm. The idea is that if you lift your elbow, the egg will drop out, thereby breaking. And if you hold your elbows too low, squeezing the egg too tightly, it will also break. Whereas such an image might help beginners, it requires the continued use of the analytical mind to decide whether the egg will fall or be crushed. Anyway, the image breaks down for moves like "White Crane" and "Four Corners." There is no way that these very-open movements can be properly done without the egg dropping.

Instead, it is much more fruitful to feel the effects of varying degrees of opening and closing and the feeling of maximizing *qi* and expansive strength.

Validating Your Progress

After learning the movements of the empty-hand Taiji form fairly accurately, a student might ask, "What's next?" Aside from learning push-hands and other forms (sword, broadsword, staff, two-person, corner operations), a very important facet is acquiring the correct internal state. But how can students know that they have achieved that state? The feeling of exhilaration and flow of *qi* are very important but not a sufficient criterion for knowing that you are on the right track. There are many things that feel good that are not Taiji or do not fit the principles. Explanations of certain internal states are like communicating what salt tastes like to someone who has never tasted it. In order to transcend such limitations, it is, therefore, necessary to have some down-to-earth criteria for evaluating your progress:

It Agrees with What Your Teacher Says and Does

This criterion has some value, but it is limited. The teacher may be withholding critical information or not explaining it clearly. Moreover, the teacher may be showing and explaining movements in a manner that facilitates learning them at the expense of transmitting important details or principles. These details might or might not be taught at a later date. Even if the information is ideally transmitted, students may not fully understand it, and they may incorrectly believe that they know what the teacher is doing in his or her movements. Physical contact with the teacher's arms and body in doing push-hands is very important in capturing a feeling of his or her internal state.

It Agrees with What Is Written in The Taiji Classics

The Taiji Classics are writings by masters over the centuries. The goal was to preserve the essential elements of Taiji for present and future *inner* students yet hide the real meanings from outsiders.

Thus, reading the Taiji Classics is more a test of your understanding than a way of learning new concepts. If you understand what was written, then you are probably on the right track. So your ability to increasingly understand what is being communicated by the Classics is a valuable sign of your progress in the art. And the parts that are still confusing are signals that more work is required.

It should be kept in mind that the Classics were written in old Chinese, then translated into modern Chinese, and then into English for those not fluent in Chinese. Therefore, there can be translation errors or misunderstandings based on the skill level of the translator(s). Nevertheless, the Classics and their elucidation are of great value and should be read and periodically reread by all Taiji practitioners regardless of level.

Your Movements Are in Accord with the Taiji Principles and Philosophy

The extent to which the principles and philosophy are expressed in the movements of the form is an indication that the corresponding inner state is correct. The main elements are balance of *yin* and *yang*, being in the moment, circularity, continuity, release of contractive muscular action, and an ability to manifest expansive strength.

You Can Use It Successfully in Push-Hands and Martial Applications

It takes a lot of skill to be able to do push-hands effectively with the correct Taiji principles, and it is fairly easy to "win" by using speed, techniques, rooting and resisting, blocking, and contractive strength. Some who practice that way feel quite virtuous and are often closed to any advice that runs counter to their accustomed modality. Similar statements apply to self-defense.

Everything Fits Together in a Satisfying Manner

As one progresses in practicing correctly and learning Taiji, its pieces increasingly fit together like those of a complex jigsaw puzzle.

The Movements Reveal Their Meaning to You

Of the myriad ways of moving in the form and push-hands, the shape of your arms, the distance of your limbs from your body, the relative timing of your arms and legs to that of the shifting and turning of your body, and the timing and continuity of stepping increasingly reveal how they should be done.

You Are Increasingly Able to Answer Your Own Questions

Without asking others, your understanding of fine points emerges and is based on the principles of naturalness, non-action, non-attachment, non-intention, being in the moment, continuity, circularity, and body unification.

Conclusion

As more of the above and possibly other ways of confirming your understanding fall into place, you can have more certainty that you are on the right track.

Chapter 16
Perspectives on Taiji

Internal Versus External Martial Arts

There are two distinctions between external and internal: (1) External martial arts were brought in from outside of China, and internal arts originated within China. (2) External arts emphasize speed, strength, and technique, and internal arts emphasize sensitivity to and understanding of force and minimal use of it.

Taijiquan, Baguazhang, and Xing-Yi Quan are examples of internal arts in both of the above senses. Ninjutsu, which is from Japan, is internal in the sense that it emphasizes sensitivity and understanding and minimal use of force.

Examples of arts that emphasize speed, strength, and technique are Shaolin (China), Karate (Japan), and Tae Kwon Do (Korea). Those studying such arts practice strikes, kicks, ground maneuvers, weapons, etc., to the point where these actions become totally automatic and dependable.

Whereas strength and speed are of value in internal arts, they are not emphasized for their own sake but as byproducts of practice of correct body usage. Techniques are not practiced in internal arts. Instead, "applications" are studied—not for the purpose of using them reflexively but for understanding and inculcating their underlying principles of action. The primary idea is to understand force and intention; that is, an opponent's touch enables an internal practitioner to be aware of the opponent's various bodily tensions and, from that, to know what the opponent wants to do next. Even without utilizing bodily contact or use of eyes, a trained internal-arts practitioner can pick up not only the opponent's intention to do harm but also the mental changes the opponent experiences as he proceeds in his attack (see discussion about *sakki* in Chapter 14).

Such knowledge of the opponent's thought process reduces the internal practitioner's need to emphasize strength and speed, which are superseded by a refinement of the timing and precision of defensive and attacking movements. For example, by the internal practitioner moving only just before the opponent's attack lands, the attacker becomes overconfident. Moreover, when a counterattack is timed right, it has a much more devastating effect.

> It is said, "If others don't move, I don't move. If others move slightly, I move first."[1]

> —Wu Yu-hsiang

Thus, practice of internal arts emphasizes cultivating sensitivity to move-ment, tension, and intention in oneself—in order to know these states of another, it is first necessary to know and be able to adjust one's own corre-sponding states. By your doing so, the opponent has a harder time reading your tensions and intention and is thereby not alerted to your actions.

To this end, movements are practiced using maximum relaxation and minimum strength, feeling everything within and without (inertia, gravity, momentum, natural swing of arms and legs). Also, when doing Push-Hands, which is a sensitivity exercise involving a partner, it is important to distinguish *yin* and *yang* (permitting your partner to enter your space without interference) and have no movements resulting from preconceived ideas.

Lifting Versus Lowering

Is lifting an arm at constant speed harder than lowering it at constant speed? Or are the two actions the same? First consider (a) holding an inanimate weight, (b) lifting it at constant speed, and (c) lowering it at constant speed (Fig. 16-1).

Let us attempt to analyze this puzzle, in terms of physics, physiology, and psychology.

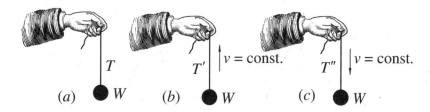

Fig. 16-1. Hand holding a string connected to a weight W (a) stationary, (b) lifting at constant speed v, and (c) lowering at constant speed v. The respective tensions in the string are T, T', and T'' (see Chapter 9 for the definition of *tension*).

---

1. Benjamin Pang Jeng Lo, Martin Inn, Robert Amacker, and Susan Foe, eds., *The Essence of T'ai Chi Ch'uan, The Literary Tradition* (Berkeley, CA: North Atlantic Books, 1985), 57.

Question 1: When the hand lifts the weight at a constant rate, is the tension T' in the string greater than, less than, or the same as the tension T when the weight is held stationary?

Question 2: When the hand lowers the weight at a constant rate, is the tension T'' in the string greater than, less than, or the same as the tension T when the weight is held stationary?

In Terms of Physics

Most people untrained in physics will intuitively think that when the weight is raised at constant speed, T' is greater than T, and when the weight is lowered at constant speed, T'' is less than T. Actually, the tension in the string is the same in all three cases. It is a consequence of Newton's first law that a mass will remain stationary or move at constant speed in a straight line only if the net force on it is zero. Thus, the downward force of gravity (its weight), which is the same in all three cases, must be balanced by the same upward pull of the string.

Note, however, that if the weight were accelerated (Fig. 16-2), the intuitive guess would be correct. That is, if the weight were accelerated upward, then T' *would* be greater than T, and if the weight were accelerated downward, then T'' *would* be less than T (Fig. 16-2).

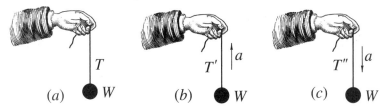

(a) T W *(b)* T' $\vert a$ W *(c)* T'' $\vert a$ W

Fig. 16-2. Hand holding a string connected to a weight W (a) stationary, (b) lifting it with an upward acceleration a, and (c) lowering it with a downward acceleration a. The respective tensions in the string are T, T', and T''.

Of course, lifting and lowering an arm differ from the actions in the examples above because an arm has leverage that changes from essentially zero when it is hanging to a maximum when it is held horizontally. As arms are raised from hanging to horizontal, the required strength increases. The opposite occurs during lowering. But the amount of strength is the same for small upward and downward excursions at a given arm level when lifting or lowering at constant speed.

In Terms of Psychology

Why then might it seem easier to lower an arm than raise it? Perhaps that perception occurs because we all know that gravity pulls massive objects downward. So, psychologically, we believe that lowering a limb is easier than raising it, and we then perceive it to be that way.

In Terms of Physiology

Even though the force required might be the same in lifting and lowering an arm at constant speed, there is a difference between how muscles are used in lifting and lowering when contractive strength is employed. When an arm is lifted, nerve impulses are sent to the muscles in the arm, shoulder, and other regions of the body to contract and shorten. But when an arm is lowered, nerve impulses are also sent to the muscles in the arm, shoulders, and other regions of the body to contract—but as the weight is lowered, these muscles are *lengthening.* The latter action involves what is called *eccentric contraction,* which is often a cause of injury. That may be why weightlifters tend to drop weights onto a wooden platform provided for that purpose instead of lowering them. Also, those with knee problems know that going up a flight of stairs is less painful than going down.

Now the question arises of how the above conclusions might differ when using expansive strength. According to our interpretation (Chapter 2), such strength results from the change in state of water in our tissues when energized by bioelectricity evoked by our intention. For use of expansive strength, there should be no difference in feeling at each point between lifting and lowering an arm at a constant rate.

Empty/Full, Yin/Yang Paradox

In Taiji, we refer to the 100-percent-weighted leg as full and the other, suspended leg as empty. By empty, we mean empty of any support of bodily weight. By full, we mean that the full weight of the body is supported by that leg.

A test of whether a leg is empty or not is to put the foot in question on a piece of thin paper. If another person can easily withdraw the paper without any resistance, then that leg is empty.

More than once in Taiji discussions, the characterization of a foot as being empty has led to a perplexing discussion of *yin* and *yang.* It goes like this: the empty foot in a 100-percent stance exerts no pressure on the floor. The fully weighted foot is supportive, earthy, inactive, and, therefore, *yin.* The empty foot is potentially ready to step or kick in an upward, outward, expansive action. Thus, the empty foot is *yang.*

However, if something is empty (insubstantial), one would think it is *yin*—not *yang.* To resolve this seeming contradiction, consider the following examples.

Imagine two balloons, one empty (inactive, yielding, lying down, soft) and the other one full of hot air (expansive, convex, firm, hot, upward). Clearly, the empty one would be *yin,* and the full one would be *yang.*

By contrast, consider two buckets, one empty, the other one full of ice water (heavy, cold). In this case, the empty bucket would be *yang* compared to the one that is full.

Thus, if we say something is empty—or any other characteristic—we can't say whether it is *yin* or *yang* without knowing the underlying conditions. *Empty* can be either *yin* or *yang*, and the context and meaning are the determining factors.

When it is said that a foot is empty, it just means that it has no weight on it and that it is potentially active and ready to step or kick ("motor running"), which is *yang*, not *yin*.

Another possible reason for confusion is that a 100-percent-weighted foot involves stretching of the quadriceps, which involves a high degree of tension. That tension is not active but passive— from totally releasing contraction and giving in to gravity. There is, however, a dot of *yang* in the *yin*, namely an upward expansion (in Taiji, nothing should ever be completely *yin* or *yang*).

Some Variations of the Taiji Symbol

In Figures 16-3 to 16-6, the correctness of the Taiji symbol is not determined by whether it appears to rotate clockwise or counterclockwise. However, the ones in Figures 16-5 and 16-6 have dark (*yin*) at the top and light (*yang*) at the bottom. These variations portray a *yin/yang* inconsistency and would be considered to be philosophically incorrect because down and dark are yin and up and light are yang, and these respective qualities should match.

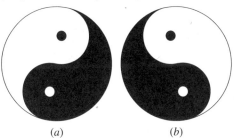

(*a*) (*b*)

Fig. 16-3. Two most-familiar variants of the Taiji symbol. These variants are philosophically correct because they have maximum *yin* at the bottom. (*a*) Clockwise and (*b*) counterclockwise.

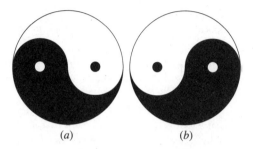

Fig. 16-4. Two less-familiar variants of the Taiji symbol. These variants are philosophically correct because they have maximum *yin* at the bottom. (*a*) Clockwise and (*b*) counterclockwise.

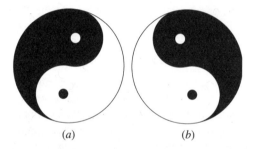

Fig. 16-5 Two philosophically incorrect variants of the Taiji symbol (maximum *yang* at bottom). (*a*) Clockwise and (*b*) counterclockwise.

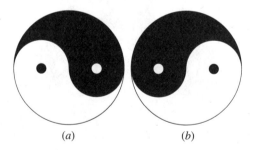

Fig. 16-6. Two philosophically incorrect variants of the Taiji symbol (maximum *yang* at bottom). (*a*) Clockwise and (*b*) counterclockwise.

Taiji "Weapons"

Many martial arts schools teach the use of sword, broadsword, staff, spear, butterfly knives, tunfa, nunchaku, etc. Whereas these traditional weapons are no longer used for self-defense, they are valuable as tools for inculcating principles of movement. A similar reason applies to Taiji sword, staff, and broadsword.

Some of the Benefits of Learning Taiji Sword

As in the empty-hand Taiji form, the Taiji sword form involves a series of continuous, relaxed, and flowing movements. There is also a two-person aspect of Taiji sword, namely, fencing, in which partners' swords continually make light contact with each other (as do the hands in push-hands practice) until a "cut" is made—ideally with just a harmless touch of a dull edge on your partner's wrist.

Practice of Taiji sword is mainly for learning the basic concepts of Taoism. The second movement in the Taiji sword form is named "The Immortal Points the Way." The immortal is Chang San-feng (1247–?),[2] the legendary originator of Taijiquan. "The Way" is the *Tao*. Thus, by practicing Taiji sword, one can directly experience and manifest the precepts of Taoism.

One of the main concepts of Taiji is non-intention, and the motion of the sword is natural rather than contrived. So once the sword movements have been learned, the sword "tells" you how to move it rather than the other way around.

The sword, which is inanimate (made of wood or unsharpened metal), should move naturally as if it were a living part of the body. The added weight, rotational inertia, linear and angular momentum, and centrifugal effect resulting from the sword's mass and spatial extension provide increased awareness of how the sword moves your body. That awareness can reveal how your limbs also do so in empty-hand movement. The sensitivity and understanding of natural movement and timing acquired through practice of Taiji sword can then carry through to elements in the empty-hand form.

A valuable feature of Taiji sword is its spirited and light footwork. Much of the stepping is preceded by successive heel and ball pivoting, which promote a feeling of almost being airborne. The result is that the movements naturally initiate from the feet to the legs and then migrate to the pelvis, through the trunk, and out from the arms, eventually reaching the tip of the sword. Over time, the turning of the trunk of the body becomes optimally timed to the circular movement of the arms and sword in a way that maximizes the transfer of motion with the least effort.

Why Taiji Sword Should Be Taught Earlier-On

Most martial arts are structured to teach empty-hand combat first even though weapons such as sticks and stones preceded empty-hand combat. The reasoning

---

2. Legend has it that Chang San-feng lived for eight hundred years and had a pet ape whom he taught to do Taijiquan and collect firewood.

is that using a weapon without a basic knowledge of self-protection will likely result in it being taken from you and used against you. But most of the weapons taught are outmoded and no longer utilized for self-protection. Also, many who study Taiji do not regard it as martial training and do not pursue learning sword, which they associate with combat. Then, when sword is taught, such instruction is usually made available only to advanced students. The result is that most Taiji practitioners are not exposed to and do not experience natural energetics of movement that can be transferred to the less-spirited empty-hand form.

Slow, meditative, empty-hand movement certainly has its value, and weapons forms are difficult to learn right away. But solely practicing empty-hand movement for too long makes it hard to break the habit of anticipating and overemphasizing "landmarks" within transitions and at the final postures. Students then tend to ignore natural movement and use muscle to get limbs to reach landmarks at the "right time." But the principles of continuous, unbroken, natural movement and timing discussed in Chapters 9 to 12 are important to incorporate into the empty-hand form as soon as the movements have been memorized and before bad habits become set. Learning sword early-on is a way to provide these benefits.

Because exposure to weapons forms is so important for enhancing natural movement, teaching sword and other weapons should occur as early as possible. That way the elements of natural movement provided can more readily carry over to the empty-hand form.

Misinterpretations

The Head Does Not Turn in Doing Taiji

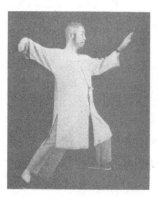

Fig. 16-7. Professor Cheng in "Single Whip."[3]

---

3. Cheng Man-ch'ing, *Tai Chi Chuan: A Simplified Method of Calisthenics for Health and Self Defense* (Berkeley, CA: North Atlantic Books, 1985), 49.

I heard this admonition applied to the Cheng Man-ch'ing style when I was a beginner at the Shi Zhong school. As with other such admonitions, which are not meant to be taken literally, this one makes no literal sense because the head unquestionably turns in space. So instead, it must mean that the head does not turn relative to the body (nose and navel always line up). Anyway, neither of these interpretations holds. For example, in the "Single Whip" posture, the head points directly west,[4] and in the immediately following posture, "Raise Hands," the head points directly north. So the transition from "Single Whip" to "Raise Hands" involves a 45-degree rotation of the torso but a 90-degree rotation of the head (see Figs. 16-7 and 16-8 for photos of Professor Cheng in the successive postures "Single Whip" and "Raise Hands"). So here, the head turns 90 degrees in space and 45 degrees relative to the body.

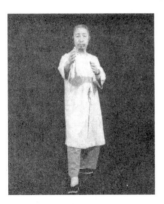

Fig. 16-8. Professor Cheng in the very next posture, "Raise Hands." Note that his head faces in the direction of the stance and has turned 90 degrees whereas the navel has turned only 45 degrees.[5]

Note that in other Taiji styles and various interpretations of them, there are other ways that the head points in final stances and moves or not during transitions.

But the admonition that the head doesn't turn may have a meaningful interpretation. Just as "a hand is not a hand" (Chapter 14) or, as sometimes stated, "The hands don't move in Taiji," have meaning only if not taken literally, perhaps "the head does not turn" should be treated likewise. Maybe what is meant is that when the head *does* turn, it doesn't turn in a haphazard, discontinuous manner. Any discontinuity in movement suggests that the mind has strayed from the present, and contraction, not expansion, is being used to turn the head. For those who have this habit of turning the head unevenly, it may be worthwhile to try the neck-relaxation exercise (Experiment 6-5), the

4. As noted previously, the starting direction is arbitrarily taken to be north.
5. Cheng, *T'ai Chi Chuan*, 51.

wrist-turning exercise (Experiment 2-4), and the soft-vision exercises (Experiments 7-12 to 7-14). The feeling of those exercises should then be applied to the turning of the head in the appropriate places in the Taiji form.

Nose and Navel

Another misinterpretation shared by some practitioners of the Cheng Man-ch'ing style is that the nose and navel always point in the same direction. Actually, the unchanging nose-navel relationship only applies to 70-30 stances and transitions between them. For 100-percent stances, the nose and forward foot point in the direction of the stance.

For a 100-percent stance with the rear foot at 90 degrees, it is impossible for the navel to point in the direction of the stance (90 degrees from the rear foot) without a damaging femuroacetabular impingement, a pathological condition in which the femur (thigh bone) exceeds its physiological range of motion and harmfully impinges on the pelvis.

Instead of pointing 90 degrees from the centerline of the rear foot, the navel naturally points midway (45 degrees) between the centerline of the rear foot and the direction of the stance. The head (nose) always points in the direction of the stance (forward foot). So, assuming that the starting direction is north, in "Raise Hands," the head and (empty) right foot point north, the left foot points west, and the navel points northwest, midway between the directions of his rear and forward feet (see Fig. 16-8 for a photo of Professor Cheng in that stance).

For what appears to be the more-recent Yang style, where the 100-percent-weighted rear foot is at 45 degrees to the direction of the stance,[6] the nose and navel *can* point in the direction of the forward foot.

Self-Defense

In my Taiji travels, I have heard that regularly practicing form and push-hands will enable you to respond appropriately in a self-defense situation just by "sinking your *qi* to your *dan tian*."

Sinking your *qi* might work in some situations but not others. If you lack extensive martial-arts training with a skilled teacher, other situations can involve trusting to luck or resorting to covering your face and pleading with the attacker not to hurt you. Muggings tend to be done from behind, by surprise, and by two or three streetwise attackers working in unison. Once you are on the ground, in pain and shock, and possibly with tears in your eyes and your own urine in your clothing, then try sinking your *qi* to your *dan tian* and see if it will work.

---

6. See www.chuckrowtaichi.com/CMCvsYang.html for a discussion of the differences between Cheng Man-ch'ing's short form and the Yang-Style long form.

Some predators utilize knives or firearms. Few Taiji experts have knowledge of how firearms function, what they can do at different distances, and how and when to defend against them—especially when not armed with an appropriate counter-tool. Even if able to disarm a predator who is wielding a handgun, some experienced martial-arts practitioners lack proper training in the use of such a tool and are unaware of the legal and civil ramifications that are likely to ensue.[7]

The Yang Long Form and Professor Cheng's Short Form

Advantages and Disadvantages of So Few/So Many Movements

In my experience, teaching the Cheng Man-ch'ing form (CMC form) allows instilling principles at an earlier stage without becoming bogged down with teaching a lot of new movements. Nevertheless, I am convinced of the benefit of teaching students the Yang long form (Yang form) after they have become proficient at the CMC form. In a self-defense situation, the subconscious mind must process a large amount of sensory information over an extended period of time, and the conscious mind is far too slow and limited to do so. The Yang form trains the subconscious mind to encompass a large number of movements, with repetitions of certain movements in different successions. For example, in the CMC form, "Single Whip" transitions into "Raise Hands," "Four Corners," and "Downward Single Whip" (two times). By comparison, in the Yang form, "Single Whip" transitions into those same movements plus "Cloud Hands" (three times) and "High Pat on Horse" (two times). Thus, the Yang form has about twice as many transitions from "Single Whip"; this presents quite a challenge to the mind not to drift, which is important in self-defense and especially in today's world.

"Brush Knee (L)" is another example of a posture leading to multiple transitions. In the CMC form, "Brush Knee (L)" transitions into "Hands Playing the Pipa," "Punch," and "Brush Knee (R)." In the Yang form, however, "Brush Knee (L)" transitions into "Hands Playing the Pipa" (two times), "Chop with Fist," "Needle at Sea Bottom" (two times), "Brush Knee (R)" (two times), and "Downward Punch." Thus, the Yang form has eight transitions from "Brush Knee (L)" compared to three such transitions in the CMC form.

---

7. See, for example, Carl Brown, *The Law and Martial Arts* (Santa Clarita, CA: Ohara Publications, Inc., 1998).

Will Practicing a Shortened Form Make You Sick?

Erle Montaigue (1949–2011) wrote in an article entitled "The Harm of Shortened Forms" that practicing a shortened form can make you sick. In that article, Montaigue says:

> I hear from so many who have been practicing shortened forms of [Taiji] for many years who are beginning to get ill for no apparent reason. Then when I tell them about shortened forms and why they shouldn't do them, they begin one of the original longer forms and hey ho, they get well again.[8]

The anecdotal nature of the above cause-and-effect assertion is problematic. It involves no scientific reasoning and provides no mechanism. That two things occurred together is insufficient for concluding that one caused the other. Was the changeover to an original, longer form with the same teacher? What other changes did the students make? How many shortened-form students become ill and recover without ever changing forms? How many longer-form students become ill and then recover after changing to a shortened form? Many people the world over get ill "for no apparent reason" and then recover without ever doing any Taiji at all! So there is no reason to think that a shortened form would make anyone sick.

The Popularization of Taiji

Yang Cheng-fu related that Yang Lu-chan, his grandfather and originator of the Yang style, took him aside and told him that he wanted him to widely popularize Taiji, not mainly for combat but to improve the failing health of his nation.[9] Yang Cheng-fu is said to have been impressed by his grandfather's wish and sought to spread Taiji.

Whereas Yang Cheng-fu taught many students, his ability to spread Taiji was limited by his inability to read or write. Thus, he encouraged literate students of his to transcribe his teachings and write books that would help spread Taijiquan.[10] Chen Wei-ming (1881–1958), a senior classmate of Cheng Man-ch'ing under Yang Cheng-fu, and Cheng Man-ch'ing did so.[11]

---

8. www.taijiworld.com/shortened-forms.html.

9. Interestingly, Yang Lu-chan (1799–1873) died about a decade before Yang Cheng-fu (1883–1936) was born. Perhaps there is a rational way of explaining how Yang Lu-chan personally communicated his wishes to his grandson consistent with this chronology.

10. Yang Chengfu, *The Essence and Applications of Taijiquan*, trans. Louis Swaim (Berkeley, CA: Blue Snake Press, 2005), 7–10.

11. Douglas Wile, comp. and trans., *T'ai Chi Touchstones: Yang Family Secret Transmissions* (Brooklyn, NY: Sweet Ch'i Press, 1983), 153–156.

When Professor Cheng came to America and saw how eager his first students were to learn, he realized that introducing Taiji to America would help fulfill his teacher's wish. At one point he said to us, "The future of Taiji is in America."

Cheng Man-ch'ing's way of spreading Taiji and making it accessible to many was to teach students the fundamentals in a pure, standardized, and simplified manner, thereby enabling his students to go on to teach in the same way. At Professor Cheng's Shi Zhong school in the 1970s, the first- and second-tier students were encouraged to teach or assist in teaching beginners' classes. Some of these students also taught Taiji outside Shi Zhong and eventually started their own schools. There was even a process at Shi Zhong for training and certifying students to teach and for then supporting them afterward. In this way, Cheng beautifully succeeded in spreading Taiji, as evidenced by the current popularity of his form and of Taiji in general.

Professor Cheng occasionally alluded to the martial or advanced internal aspects of Taiji (see Chapter 3, "Swimming on Land"). But he did not emphasize or teach these aspects, which is certainly understandable. He must have assumed that after he was gone, his direct students would naturally find other teachers who would enable them to advance. But few of them pursued other teachers or learned other styles or advanced modalities of Taiji movement. Moreover, some of Professor Cheng's students felt that changing anything they were taught by him would be disrespectful, which is ironic because Professor Cheng made a number of changes to what he was taught. In fact, some feel that he created a separate style.[12,13]

At present, the Cheng Man-ch'ing form comprises a very clearly defined way of teaching and moving. Most practitioners of that form have softness—an essential first stage—but tend to lack internal strength, an element also emphasized by Yang Cheng-fu. As Yang said, "Taijiquan is the art of concealing hardness in softness, like a needle in cotton."[14] So softness is necessary—but it is not sufficient.

12. See Master Koh Ah-tee interviewed by Nigel Sutton of the Zhong Ding Traditional Chinese Martial Arts Association, http://wuweitaichi.com/articles/Master_Koh_Ah_Tee.htm.

13. For occurrences and comparisons of movements in both the Yang and Cheng Man-ch'ing forms, visit https://www.chuckrowtaichi.com/CMCvsYang.html.

14. *T'ai Chi Touchstones: Yang Family Secret Transmissions*, p. 3.

AFTERWORD

Through teaching and writing over the decades, I have learned greatly from sharing my knowledge of Taiji, Qigong, nutrition, the prenatal origin of music, and the historical tuning of keyboard instruments. I have also experienced much fulfillment from knowing that I have enriched others in doing so. Such was my motivation for writing this book.

My goal is not just to help fellow practitioners and teachers; it is also to enable Taiji to be more of what it should and can be. Important elements have been removed from Taiji and too often are not taught, not because of their intrinsic difficulty but because they have been concealed for centuries, making them difficult to grasp and transmit. My approach to unraveling and articulating some of the obscure Taiji concepts has involved applying what I have learned from my studies of diverse disciplines such as Kinetic Awareness®, physics, philosophy, and other internal martial arts such as Baguazhang, I Liq-chuan, and Ninjutsu.

The main thrust of this book involves essentially two dimensions. One dimension is expansive strength, which is often described enigmatically as *qi* or mind. Whereas I have not yet encompassed the full scientific underpinnings of this dimension, what I have provided is a start, which others will take further. The second dimension is the timing of the movement of the pelvis relative to that of the hands to maximize the transfer of movement from the ground through the body and out. These two dimensions are natural but easily overlooked and often misunderstood.

It is my hope that the remainder of the contents of the book will also provide value, and I have tried to clearly represent them in a manner that is not otherwise readily available. I have purposely left out what is clearly explained elsewhere. And I have included only subject matter that I have experienced over sufficient time to be satisfied that it is consistent with the spirit of the Taiji Classics and matches what highly skilled Taiji practitioners display and seek to transmit.

I also hope this book will prompt others to further clarify the hidden concepts in Taiji and make them more accessible.

ACKNOWLEDGMENTS

I am indebted to my teachers, especially Cheng Man-ch'ing, William C. C. Ch'en, Elaine Summers, Alice Holtman, Harvey Sober, Kevin Harrington, and Sam Chin Fan-siong. I am also indebted to my classmates and my students. All of these people have immensely contributed to my education and development.

Sensei Peter Doherty's knowledge as a trainer has contributed greatly to my understanding of expansive strength and, especially, its use in improving spine alignment. I am grateful to Chip Carter, Michael Ehrenreich, Gregory Falkin, Jo Ann Tannenbaum, Robert Tipp, Paul Wood, and Alan Zimmerman for making suggestions and pointing out errors in early drafts of the book. Robert Tipp was especially helpful in researching and elucidating the included Chinese characters. I thank Ed Young for explaining the meanings of the primeval characters for *Shí Zhòng*, used by Professor Cheng Man-ch'ing in naming his Taiji school. I also thank my wife, Ruth Baily, for her frequent help with word usage.

I am grateful to David Ripianzi for his guidance and advice regarding the manner of presentation of concepts and to Leslie Takao for her excellent editing skills. I also thank copy editor Doran Hunter whose knowledge and amazing skill and perseverance at finding and suggesting ways of improving clarity have significantly enhanced this book.

I thank Ruth Baily, Michael Dimeo, Peter Doherty, Kenneth Van Sickle, JoAnn Tannenbaum, and Alan Zimmerman for taking photographs. I also thank Ellen Cheng for permitting use of photos of her father, Cheng Man-ch'ing.

I am especially grateful to Peter Varley of the UK, who suggested that I contact Dr. Gerald Pollack of Washington State University. Pollack's research on water and cells provided a viable mechanism for explaining expansive strength. And, of course, I am quite grateful to Dr. Pollack for his work and willingness to answer my questions in that regard.

Appendix 1
Supplement to Chapters 8 and 9

Basics of Vector Addition

In order to analyze rooting and the swing of limbs, we must take into account the combined effects of the different forces involved. Elementary physics provides the tools for dealing with such effects through the use of vectors. Thus, we will first explain the nature of vector quantities and how they are added.

Vectors

Distinction between Scalars and Vectors

In basic physics, we encounter two different kinds of quantities, scalars and vectors. Scalars can be specified by just a number (magnitude alone). Vectors are specified by magnitude and direction. Examples of scalars and vectors are listed in Table A1-1.

Scalars (Magnitude Only)	Vectors (Magnitude and Direction)
time	
mass	
speed	velocity
temperature	
length	displacement
area	
volume	
	force
	weight

Table A1-1. List of scalar and vector counterparts of some physical quantities. Note that the weight of an object is the force of gravity on it. Thus weight has a direction (toward the center of the earth) and is, therefore, technically a vector. Additionally, length is the scalar counterpart of displacement, which is a vector. Time and mass have no vector counterparts.

In our analysis, we will be dealing with forces in different directions, and it will be necessary to add their effects using vectors. Therefore, a basic treatment of vectors is next provided.

Representing a Vector

To represent a vector quantity, we draw an arrow whose direction is that of the quantity and whose length is proportional to its magnitude. In printed matter, a vector is labeled in bold type ($\mathbf{V}$), and by hand, it is written with an arrow on top ($\overrightarrow{V}$).

Adding Vectors

To add two vectors, we place the tail of one vector on the head of the other. The sum $\mathbf{V_1} + \mathbf{V_2}$ (called the resultant $\mathbf{R}$) goes from the tail of $\mathbf{V_1}$ to the head of $\mathbf{V_2}$. For example, consider adding $\mathbf{V_1}$ = 3 miles east and $\mathbf{V_2}$ = 4 miles north (Fig. A1-1).

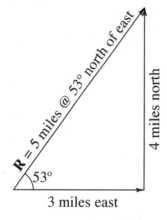

Fig. A1-1. The addition of two perpendicular vectors.

Order of Adding Vectors

Note that the order of adding vectors does not matter; namely,
$\mathbf{V_1} + \mathbf{V_2} = \mathbf{V_2} + \mathbf{V_1}$, as shown in Figure A1-2.

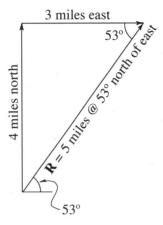

3 miles east

53°

53° north of east

4 miles north

$R = 5$ miles @ 53° north of east

53°

Fig. A1-2. The addition of the vectors in Fig A1-1 added in a different order gives the same resultant; namely, where you end up is independent of which leg of the trip occurs first.

Components of a Vector

When adding vectors that are not mutually perpendicular, the Pythagorean theorem and simple trigonometry are insufficient. In that case, we utilize the components of the vectors. The components of a vector are scalars found by drawing a perpendicular line from the vector's head to each of the coordinate axes (Fig. A1-3). The components are the "shadows" of the vector on the coordinate axes.

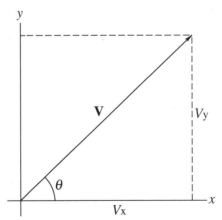

Fig. A1-3. The x and y components V_x and V_y of a vector **V**.

Vector Addition Using Components

To add two or more vectors **A**, **B**, **C**, . . ., break them down into their x and y components. Then the x and y components R_x and R_y of the resultant **R** are:

$$R_x = A_x + B_x + C_x + \ldots$$
$$R_y = A_y + B_y + C_y + \ldots$$
$$R^2 = R_x^2 + R_y^2$$

and $\tan \theta = R_y/R_x$.

Example. Using components, add vectors **A** and **B**, where **A** = 3 ∡ 0° and **B** = 4 ∡ 90°.

Solution.

$$A_x = 3 \cos 0° = 3\ (1) = 3,$$
$$A_y = 3 \sin 0° = 3\ (0) = 0,$$
$$B_x = 4 \cos 90° = 4\ (0) = 0,$$
$$B_y = 4 \sin 90° = 4\ (1) = 4.$$
$$R_x = A_x + B_x = 3 + 0 = 3,$$
$$R_y = A_y + B_y = 0 + 4 = 4,$$
$$R^2 = 3^2 + 4^2 = 9 + 16 = 25,$$
$$R = 5.$$
$$\tan \theta = R_y/R_x = 4/3 = 1.33,$$
$$\theta = 53.13°.$$

Answer: R = 5 ∡ 53.13° (as we saw in Fig. A1-2).

Torque

Torque is a quantity that is a measure of the rotational effect of a force about a point. Torque is represented by the Greek letter τ. The torque τ_Q of a force **F** about a point Q is found by first drawing a line l from Q to **F** (Fig. A1-4).

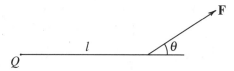

Fig. A1-4. To find the torque of a force **F** about a point Q, a line is drawn from Q to **F**.

The magnitude of the torque of **F** about Q is found by multiplying l by the component of **F** perpendicular to l, namely, $\tau_Q = lF \sin \theta$. Note that the component of **F** parallel to l has no rotational effect (Fig. A1-5). The torque of a force is considered to be negative if its rotational effect is clockwise, and it is considered to be positive if its rotational effect is counterclockwise. The torque of **F** in Figure A1-6 is, therefore, $\tau_Q = + lF \sin \theta$.

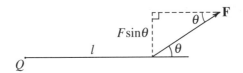

Fig. A1-5. The broken lines represent the perpendicular and parallel components of a force **F** with respect to the line l drawn from Q to **F**.

To find the torque of a number of forces, the individual torques are added, taking into account if they are clockwise (negative) or counterclockwise (positive).

Appendix 2
Supplement to Chapter 8

Analysis of Forces in Rooting

The following analysis applies to the Rooting and Redirecting discussion of Chapter 8. The goal is to find the optimal relationships for not being moved by another's force.

Force Diagram

In the diagram in Figure A2-1, line QR, tilted with respect to the vertical at an angle θ, represents the axis of the person being pushed. The effect of the forward leg is neglected because the supportive effect of that leg disappears when the receiving person starts to lose rooting, which is the limiting case being considered. In fact, some practitioners purposely lift their forward leg off the ground while demonstrating rooting.

Assumptions

We will assume that the person being pushed is in both rotational and translational equilibrium. Then we will investigate the effects produced when different parameters are varied and draw conclusions.

For a body to be in translational equilibrium, the sum of all forces on it must equal zero. For a body to be in rotational equilibrium, the sum of the torques of all forces about any point must equal zero.

Rotational Stability

Setting the sum Σ of torques about Q equal to zero (see Fig. A2-1):

$$\Sigma \tau_Q = 0$$

$$lP \sin \phi - l'W \sin \theta = 0.$$

$$\text{Therefore, } P = \frac{l'W \sin \theta}{l \sin \phi}. \quad \text{(Eq. 1)}$$

Note that l, l', and W are constants. Thus, assuming continuing stability of the person being pushed, we will investigate the effect of different values of θ and ϕ on the magnitude P of the force exerted by the person pushing. The larger P, the greater the force exerted by the person pushing without loss of stability of the person being pushed.

Conclusions

Looking at Eq. 1, we see that as θ increases, so does P because, as θ increases from 0° to 90°, $\sin \theta$ increases from 0 to 1. Thus, extending your rear leg as far back as possible and leaning forward increases θ, thereby increasing your stability due to the effect of your weight.

Also, as ϕ increases from 0 to 90°, $\sin \phi$ increases from 0 to 1. Because $\sin \phi$ is in the denominator, the *smaller* the angle ϕ is, the *larger* the force P can be without any loss in stability of the person being pushed. In fact, as ϕ approaches zero, P approaches infinity! The extreme condition (infinite P) means that no matter how much force a person exerts on you along the line QR, your stability will be maintained.

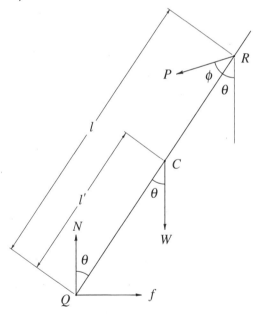

$Q =$	the center of the receiving person's rear foot
$R =$	the point of contact of the pushing person
$f =$	the force of friction of the floor on the receiving person's rear foot

$N =$	the upward force supplied by the floor
$C =$	the center of mass of the receiving person
$W =$	the force of gravity on the receiving person (his weight)
$P =$	the magnitude of the force of the person pushing
$\phi =$	the angle between the line QR and the direction of P
$\theta =$	the angle between the line QR and the vertical
$l =$	the distance from Q to R
$l' =$	the distance from Q to C

Fig. A2-1. Forces on a person who is demonstrating rooting. QR represents the line from the center of his rear foot to the point of applied force.

Friction with the Floor

The effects of W, θ, and ϕ on the frictional force f of the floor are found by setting the sum Σ of horizontal components of all forces to zero (equilibrium):

$$\Sigma F_x = 0.$$

Assuming no slipping,

$$f - P \sin (\theta + \phi) = 0$$

Therefore, $f = P \sin (\theta + \phi)$.   (Eq. 2)

Setting the vertical components of all forces to zero:

$$\Sigma F_y = 0$$

$$N - W - P \cos (\theta + \phi) = 0$$

Therefore, $N = W + P \cos (\theta + \phi)$.   (Eq. 3)

Also, the maximum frictional force is given by $f\text{max} = \mu_s N$, where μ_s is the coefficient of static (not sliding) friction between the floor and the foot of the person being pushed. μ_s depends only on the nature of the surfaces (for example, wood and rubber).

Therefore, $f_{\text{max}} = \mu_s [W + P \cos (\theta + \phi)]$.   (Eq. 4)

Conclusions

Note that cosine increases as its argument decreases. From Eq. 3, it can be seen that as θ and/or ϕ decreases, f_{max} increases. That relationship means that the more you extend your rear leg and the more along line QR you are pushed, the greater the frictional force of the floor on your rear foot and the less chance you will slide backward.

The question is how you can regulate the direction of the pusher's force to your advantage. To this end, consider next the reaction to the forces exerted by the person pushing. According to Newton's third law, if object A exerts a force on object B (the action), then B exerts an equal-and-opposite force on A (the reaction). Thus, when the person A (the person pushing) exerts a force of magnitude P in a certain direction on person B (the person receiving), then B automatically exerts a force of magnitude P on A in the opposite direction. If the force of the person pushing has a downward component, the reaction force exerted back on him will automatically have a corresponding upward component. The smaller the angle ϕ, the more B will be rooted (not losing balance or sliding) and the more A will be losing balance and sliding.

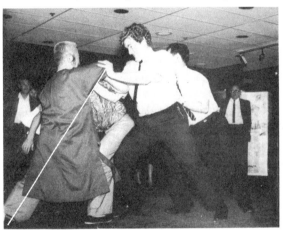

Fig. A2-2. Note that the line drawn from the center of Professor Cheng's rear foot to the point of contact of Patrick Watson is along his rear leg. Note also that Professor Cheng's right arm is pushing Watson's left arm slantingly upward, causing Watson to push Professor Cheng's arm slantingly downward.

So how can B get A to push along the line RQ ($\phi = 0$)? The answer is for B to exert an upward force on A, thereby causing A to exert a downward reaction force on B. Note in Fig. A2-2 how Professor Cheng's elbow is lifted, causing Patrick Watson to push partly downward. The combination of downward and forward forces exerted by Watson is then a single resultant force directed toward Professor Cheng's rear foot, thus causing Professor Cheng to be more rooted and less likely to slide backward but lifting Watson, causing him to be less rooted and more likely to slide backward.

Appendix 3

Supplement to Chapter 9

Analysis of Swing of Hanging Rods

Swing of Pivoted Rod When Displaced and Released (Modality 2)

We next consider a rod hanging from a frictionless pivot, displaced at an angle θ_i and then released (Fig. A3-1a). The motion of the rod should approximate that of a relaxed arm hanging from a shoulder similarly displaced. As with the simple pendulum, the rod swings to its highest level on the other side (Fig. A3-1b), making a final angle θ_f with the vertical, and continues swinging back and forth with decreasing amplitude due to friction.

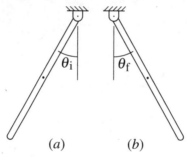

(a)   (b)

Fig. A3-1. A physical pendulum, consisting of a rod of length l, mass m, hanging from a frictionless, stationary pivot. (a) Rod is displaced so that it makes an initial angle θ_i with the vertical. (b) Rod swings to its highest on the other side, making a final angle θ_f with the vertical.

As with the simple pendulum, for the first swing, θ_f approximately equal θ_i, the amplitude of motion decreases, and the rod eventually comes to rest.

> **Experiment A3-1.** In a standing position, let your arm hang. Feel its weight, and release as much tension in your arm and shoulder as possible. Then, without moving your shoulder, have somebody lift your arm forward and release it. Note how your arm swings backward and then forward, nearly at the same height from which it started. Then it swings back and forth with decreasing amplitude until it comes to rest.

See how becoming more relaxed increases the number of swings before your arm comes to rest.

Horizontally Moving Rod After the Pivot Is Suddenly Fixed (Modality 3)

We are next interested in the swing of a hanging arm when the shoulder is moving forward (or backward) and then stops. In this regard, consider a thin rod of length $2l$, mass m, hanging from a frictionless pivot, moving at a constant horizontal velocity v_0 (Fig. A3-2a). Let A be a point at the pivot at the instant the pivot becomes fixed (Fig. A3-2b). As with the simple pendulum, for the first swing, θ_f approximately equal θ_i (Fig. A3-2c). The rod will then swing back and forth, with the amplitude of motion decreasing until it eventually comes to rest.

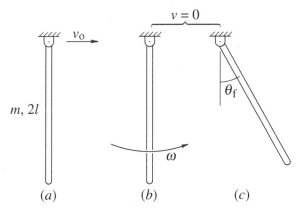

Fig. A3-2. (a) Rod of mass m, length $2l$ (to simplify calculations), hanging from a frictionless pivot, moving at a constant horizontal velocity v_0. (b) The pivot becomes fixed, causing the rod to have an angular velocity ω. (c) Rod swings to its highest level, making a final angle θ_f.

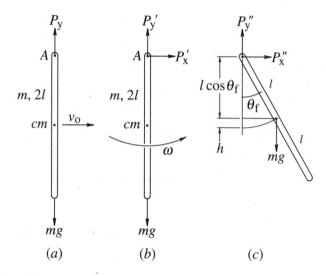

Fig. A3-3. Free-body diagrams of the rod in Figure A3-2. Such a diagram shows all forces on the rod. (a) The rod immediately before the pivot becomes fixed. (b) The rod immediately after the pivot becomes fixed. (c) The rod having swung to its greatest angle θ_f. P_x, P_x', P_x'', P_y, P_y', and P_y'' are the x and y components of the force on the rod by the pivot as the problem evolves, mg is the gravitational force on the rod, and ω is the angular velocity of the rod immediately after the pivot is fixed.

Analysis. In such problems, it is customary to draw a free-body diagram, which is a diagram showing all forces on the rod (Fig. A3-3) for each appropriate stage of the movement. Angular momentum about the pivot point A is conserved during the evolution from (a) to (b) because, as long as the rod is vertical, all forces (gravitational and other forces exerted by the pivot) go through A and, therefore, have zero torque about that point.

The rod's initial angular momentum L_A about A is mv_0l (its linear momentum multiplied by the distance from A to the rod's center of mass). Immediately after the pivot becomes fixed, the angular momentum L'_A is $I_A\omega$, where $I_A = m(2l)^2/3 = 4ml^2/3$ is the moment of inertia about A, and ω is the angular velocity of the rod just after fixing. Thus, $L'_A = 4ml^2\omega/3$. Setting the angular momentum immediately before the fixing to that immediately after, we get

$$L_A = L'_A$$

$$mv_0l = [4ml^2/3]\omega.$$

The above expression reduces to

$$\omega = 3v_0/4l.$$

Once the pivot is fixed, mechanical energy is conserved because no force other than gravity does work. Therefore, the initial kinetic energy of the rod becomes all potential energy when the rod reaches its highest angle θ_f with respect to the vertical. The kinetic energy after fixing is $I_A \omega^2/2$. The increase in potential energy when the rod reaches θ_f (kinetic energy = 0) is mgh, where $h = (l - l \cos \theta_f) = l(1 - \cos \theta_f)$. Setting the initial kinetic energy at (a) equal to the final potential energy at (c) (energy is conserved), we get

$$(4ml^2/\omega)\omega^2/2 = mgl(1 - \cos \theta_f).$$
$$(4l/3)\omega^2/2 = g(1 - \cos \theta_f).$$

Substituting the value previously found for ω, we get

$$(2l/3)(3v_0/4l)^2 = g(1 - \cos \theta_f),$$
which reduces to
$$\cos \theta_f = 1 - 3v_0^2/8gl, \text{ (Eq. 1)}$$

where g = 9.8 m/s^2 is the acceleration due to gravity. Note that the above result does not depend on the mass of the rod.

Intuitive explanation. When the pivot of the hanging rod is suddenly stopped, the top of the rod must also come to a stop. But all of the other particles of the rod have movement, which tends to continue. So the resulting motion of the rod is rotational about the pivot. However, the pull of gravity slows down the upward rotation until the rod momentarily stops and then swings backward.

The relationship to Taiji. To simulate a condition typical to Taiji movement we can estimate that a human arm has a length of about 2/3 of a meter, and the velocity of the moving shoulder is about 1/2 m/s.

Substituting v_0 = 0.5 m/s, $2l$ = 2/3 m, and g = 9.8 m/s^2 into Eq. 1, we get
$$\cos \theta_f = 1 - 3(0.5)^2/8(9.8)(1/3),$$
$$\cos \theta_f = 1 - 9(0.25)/8(9.8).$$

Solving, we get
$$\theta_f = 13.8°.$$

Experiment A3-2. Let your arm loosely hang from your shoulder while moving your shoulder forward. Then suddenly stop. Note how your arm continues to move forward. Then it will swing forward and backward with decreasing amplitude until it comes to a stop.

Swing of Frictionlessly Pivoted, Hanging, Rod When the Pivot Is Then Accelerated Horizontally (Modality 4)

Again consider a rod motionlessly hanging from a frictionless pivot, when the pivot is suddenly accelerated. The motion of the rod should approximate that of a relaxed arm hanging from a shoulder similarly accelerated (Fig. A3-4).

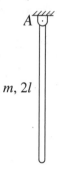

A

$m, 2l$

Fig. A3-4. A rod of length mass m, $2l$, motionlessly hanging from a frictionless pivot (point A). The pivot is then accelerated to the right with a_A.

Analysis. We will next find the motion of the hanging rod when the pivot is accelerated to the right. Refer to the free-body diagram in Figure A3-5.

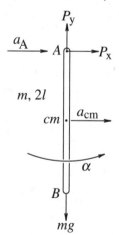

P_y

a_A A P_x

$m, 2l$

cm a_{cm}

α

B

mg

Fig. A3-5. Free-body diagram of a rod of mass m, length $2l$, hanging from a frictionless pivot, which is then accelerated to the right. Such a diagram shows all forces on the rod. P_x and P_y are the x and y components, respectively, of the force on the rod by the pivot, mg is the gravitational force on the rod, and a_{cm} is the acceleration of the center of mass. Also, points A and B are at the pivot and bottom of the rod, respectively.

The equations that will be used are $\Sigma F = ma_{cm}$ (the sum of all forces ΣF equals the acceleration $\mathbf{a}_{cm}$ of the center of mass) and $\Sigma\tau_{cm} = I_{cm}\alpha$ ($\Sigma\tau_{cm}$ is the sum of all torques about the center of mass, I_{cm} is the moment of inertia about the center of mass, and α is the angular acceleration of the rod, assumed counterclockwise).

During the moment that the rod is still vertical, it is in equilibrium in the y direction, so $P_y = mg$, and the acceleration is in the x direction. Applying Newton's second law, $\Sigma F = ma_{cm}$ in the x direction, we get:

$$P_x = ma_{cm}.$$

Applying $\Sigma\tau_{cm} = I_{cm}\alpha$ and taking counterclockwise as positive, we get:

$$-P_x l = m[(2l)^2/12]\alpha.$$

Combining the above two equations, we get:

$$-ma_{cm}\, l = (ml^2/3)\alpha.$$

Simplifying, we get:

$$a_{cm} = -l\alpha/3. \qquad \text{Eq. 1}$$

Relative acceleration:

$$a_B = a_{B/cm} + a_{cm}. \qquad \text{Eq. 2}$$

But
$$a_{B/cm} = l\alpha. \qquad \text{Eq. 3}$$

Substituting Eqs. 1 and 3 into Eq. 2, we get
$$a_B = l\alpha - l\alpha/3.$$

$$a_B = 2l\alpha/3. \qquad \text{Eq. 4}$$

Similarly,
$$a_A = a_{A/cm} + a_{cm}. \qquad \text{Eq. 5}$$

But
$$a_{A/cm} = -l\alpha. \qquad \text{Eq. 6}$$

Substituting Eqs. 1 and 6 into Eq. 5, we get
$$a_A = -l\alpha + -l\alpha/3,$$

$$a_A = -4l\alpha/3. \qquad \text{Eq. 7}$$

Comparing Eqs. 4 and 7, we see that

$$a_B = -a_A/2.$$

Conclusion. When the pivot of the rod at its top is accelerated to the right by a, the bottom is accelerated to the *left* by $a/2$.

Intuitive explanation. When the pivot of the hanging rod is suddenly moved to the right, the top of the rod must also move to the right. But all of the other particles of the rod have inertia, which results in their tending to lag behind. So the resulting motion of the rod is a backward rotation about the pivot.

BIBLIOGRAPHY

Ball, Robert. *Wonders of Acoustics*. New York: Charles Scribner & Co., 1870.

Brown, Carl. *The Law and Martial Arts*. Santa Clarita, CA: Ohara Publications, Inc., 1998.

Chen, Yearning K. *Tai-Chi Chuan: Its Effects and Practical Applications*. Van Nuys, CA: New Castle Publishing Co., 1979.

Cheng Man-ch'ing and Robert Smith. *T'ai-Chi: The "Supreme Ultimate" Exercise for Health, Sport, and Self-Defense*. Rutland, VT: Charles E. Tuttle Co., 1969.

Cheng Man-ch'ing. *Cheng Tzu's Thirteen Treatises on T'ai Chi Ch'uan*. Translated by Benjamin Pang Jen Lo and Martin Inn. Berkeley, CA: North Atlantic Books, 1981.

———. *Master Cheng's Thirteen Chapters on T'ai-Chi Ch'uan*. Translated by Prof. Douglas Wile. Brooklyn, NY: Sweet Ch'i Press, 1982.

———. *T'ai Chi Chuan: A Simplified Method of Calisthenics for Health & Self-Defense*. Richmond, VA: North Atlantic Books, 1981.

Chin, Sam F.S. *I Liq Chuan: Martial Art of Awareness*. Mount Kisco, NY: Chin Family I Liq Chuan Association, 2006.

Chuckrow, Robert. "A Biological Interpretation of Ch'i." *Qi: The Journal of Traditional Eastern Health & Fitness* 21, no. 3 (Autumn 2011).

———. "A Clarification of 'Secret' Teachings Revealed by Cheng Man-ch'ing." *Qi: The Journal of Traditional Eastern Health & Fitness* 20, no. 4 (Winter 2010).

———. "Stepping Like a Cat." *Qi: The Journal of Traditional Eastern Health & Fitness* 24, no. 3 (Autumn 2014).

———. *T'ai Chi Ch'uan: Embracing the Pearl*. Briarcliff Manor, NY: Rising Mist Publications, 1995. Republished as *The Tai Chi Book*. Boston: YMAA Publication Center, 1998.

———. *Tai Chi Dynamics*. Wolfeboro, NH: YMAA Publication Center, 2008.

———. *Tai Chi Walking*. Wolfeboro, NH: YMAA Publication Center, 2002.

———. *The Tai Chi Book*. Wolfeboro, NH: YMAA Publication Center, 1998.

Fu Zhongwen. *Mastering Yang-Style Taijiquan*. Trans. Louis Swaim. Berkeley, CA: Blue Snake Books, 2006,

Hayes, Stephen K. *The Ninja and Their Secret Fighting Art*. Rutland, VT: Charles E. Tuttle Company, 1981.

Ho, George K. W. "Going Beyond the Term Relaxation," *Tai Chi Magazine* 38, no. 1 (Spring 2014): 6–9.

LeBoyer, Frederick, *Birth Without Violence*. New York: Alfred A. Knopf, 1980.

Lee Ying-arng. *Lee's Modified Tai Chi for Health*. Honolulu: Mclisa Enterprises, 1968.

Liang, T.T. *T'ai Chi Ch'uan for Health and Self-Defense: Philosophy and Practice*. New York: Vintage Books, 1977.

Liao, Waysun. *T'ai Chi Classics*. Boston: Shambhala, 2000.

Lo, Benjamin Pang-jeng, ed. *The Essence of T'ai Chi Ch'uan, The Literary Tradition*. Berkeley, CA: North Atlantic Books, 1985.

Manser, Martin H. *Concise English-Chinese Chinese-English Dictionary*, 2nd ed. Hong Kong: Oxford University Press, 1999.

Nelson, Andrew N. *The Modern Reader's Japanese-English Character Dictionary: Original Classic*. North Clarendon, VT Tuttle Publishing, 1995.

Pollack, Gerald H. *Cells, Gels, and the Engines of Life*. Seattle: Ebner and Sons Publishing, 2001.

Pollack, Gerald H. *The Fourth Phase of Water*. Seattle: Ebner and Sons Publishing, 2013.

Shaw, Edward R. *Physics by Experiment*. New York: Maynard, Merrill, & Co., 1897.

T'ai-Chi Ch'uan, Body and Mind. New York: Tai Chi Chuan Association, 1968.

Vaccari, Oreste, and Enko Elsoa Vaccari. *Pictorial Chinese-Japanese Characters*. Rutland, VT: Charles E. Tuttle Co., 1950.

Webster's New International Dictionary of the English Language, 2nd Edition, Unabridged. Springfield, MA: G. & C. Merriam Co., 1954.

Wile, Douglas, comp and trans. *T'ai Chi Touchstones: Yang Family Secret Transmissions*. Brooklyn, NY: Sweet Ch'i Press, 1983.

Yang Chengfu. *The Essence and Applications of Taijiquan*. Translated by Louis Swaim. Berkeley: Blue Snake Books, 2005.

Zhongwen, Fu. Mastering Yang-Style Taijiquan. Translated by Louis Swaim. Berkeley, CA: Blue

INTERNET REFERENCES

Benign paroxysmal positional vertigo treatment: https://www.ncbi.nlm.nih.gov/books/NBK458287/.

Chen Shih-hsing (Chen Shixing) demonstrating T'ai-Chi applications: https://www.youtube.com/watch?v=uA-4gPb3tfo.

Chen Hsiao-wang (Chen Xiaowang) demonstrating rooting: https://www.youtube.com/watch?v=FtCfUaL-leo.

Jin, li, etc. discussion: http://www.ycgf.org/Articles/TJ_Jin/TJ_Jin1.html.

Dogs shaking off water in slow motion: https://www.youtube.com/watch?v=HVe5caFCUrE.

Elaine Summers' biography: http://en.wikipedia.org/wiki/Elaine_Summers.

Jade Belt variations (8:00-minute point): https://www.youtube.com/watch?v=bAhNA23UTeE&t=8s.

Jaguar stalking a crocodile: https://www.youtube.com/watch?v=DBNYwxDZ_pA.

Knee, ankle, and arch alignment: https://chuckrowtaichi.com/Alignment.html.

Koh Ah inte's rview: http://wuweitaichi.com/articles/Master_Koh_Ah_Tee.htm.

Krishnamurti talking about meditation: https://www.youtube.com/watch?v=Z_QpHabajKI&t=70s.

Masaaki Hatsumi testing Ninjutsu students: https://www.youtube.com/watch?v=-zNP7-unHrw and https://www.youtube.com/watch?v=i-GidagO6C8.

Mindfulness: http://www.wisebrain.org/papers/MindfulnessPsyTx.pdf.

Monkeys on typewriters: https://en.wikipedia.org/wiki/Infinite_monkey_theorem.

New organ missed by gold standard methods: https://nyulangone.org/press-releases/researchers-find-new-organ-missed-by-gold-standard-methods-for-visualizing-anatomy-disease.

Physical quantity definition: http://en.wikipedia.org/wiki/Physical_quantity/.) Some examples are length, mass, time, and speed.

Pinyin/Wade-Giles conversions: http://library.ust.hk/guides/opac/conversion-tables.html.

Protists (video): https://www.youtube.com/watch?v=4aZneo5Qu4Q and https://www.youtube.com/watch?v=-8rpGbHC2Jo.

Robert Smith: https://en.wikipedia.org/wiki/Robert_W._Smith_(writer).

Sarcomere: https://en.wikipedia.org/wiki/Sarcomere.

Shortened forms "can make you sick": www.taijiworld.com/shortened-forms.html.

Stretching routine: https://www.chuckrowtaichi.com/StretchingRoutine.html.

Structural elements of the human body are capable of transducing mechanical energy into an electric current: https://www.ncbi.nlm.nih.gov/pubmed/577004.

Taiji can improve cognitive function: https://www.health.harvard.edu/mind-and-mood/a-sharper-mind-tai-chi-can-improve-cognitive-function.

Taiji boosts brain functioning article: http://www.huffingtonpost.com/2012/06/22/tai-chi-brain-functioning-memory_n_1612276.html.

Tacoma Narrows Bridge Collapse: https://www.youtube.com/watch%3Fv%3Dj-zczJXSxnw.

Taiji's Substance & Application, translation by Paul Brennan, Sept. 2013, https://brennantranslation.wordpress.com/2013/09/14/explaining-taiji-principles-taiji-fa-shuo/?fbclid=IwAR1HUgWy-U2ekQb0u-gtYY7T6p_5JLG37-31hee53d84nBLzo7dC_i3LqCc.

Turtle Qigong: https://www.youtube.com/watch?v=ZOhoUyxIgaU.

Unusual aspects of water: https://www.youtube.com/watch?v=i-T7tCMUDXU&feature=youtu.be.

Wang Shu-chin doing T'ai-Chi form: https://www.youtube.com/watch?v=JnhEwTAQr7Q&t=177s.

Wang Shu-chin taking punches: https://www.youtube.com/watch?v=JnhEwTAQr7Q&t=489s.

Wang Shu-chin Wikipedia article: https://en.wikipedia.org/wiki/Wang_Shujin.

Winslow Homer painting: http://www.metmuseum.org/toah/works-of-art/22.220.

Yang and Cheng Man-ch'ing form comparisons: https://www.chuckrowtaichi.com/CMCvsYang.html.

Yang Lu-chan, grandfather of Yang Cheng-fu. Historical perspective and interesting stories: https://en.wikipedia.org/wiki/Yang_Luchan.

Yang Sau-chung (1910–1985), Yang Cheng-fu's first son, doing the Yang form: http://youtu.be/Bze07WyY0C0.

Yin and Yang in "Ward Off": https://www.chuckrowtaichi.com/YinYangInWardOff.mp4.

INDEX

ABOUT THE AUTHOR

Robert Chuckrow (1936–) has studied Taiji, Qigong, and other movement, self-development, and healing arts since 1970 under high-level masters such as Cheng Man-ch'ing, William C. C. Ch'en, Elaine Summers, Alice Holtman, Harvey I. Sober, Kevin Harrington, and Sam Chin Fan-siong. He has taught Taiji extensively and has authored five prior books, three on Taiji. His *The Tai Chi Book* was a finalist in the Independent Publisher Book Awards in the health/ medicine category. His book, *Tai Chi Dynamics*, won two awards: the 2008 USA Book News award for "best book in health: exercise and fitness" and the Eric Hoffer award.

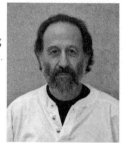

Chuckrow is certified as a master teacher of Kinetic Awareness®, has a Ph.D. in experimental physics from NYU, and has taught physics at NYU, The Cooper Union, Fieldston, and other schools.

BOOKS FROM YMAA

VIDEO FROM YMAA

more products available from . . .

YMAA Publication Center, Inc. 楊氏東方文化出版中心

1-800-669-8892 • info@ymaa.com • www.ymaa.com